CLEANSE & PURIFY
THYSELF

"and I will exalt thee to the throne of power."

by
Dr. Richard Anderson, N.D., N.M.D.

✠

Dedicated to

The Source of All Life–our Divine Mother and Father–and all the Sons of God who have purified themselves before us and have come back to help us do likewise; also to all the strong, wonderful souls who are willing to purify themselves so that they may be "rewarded openly".

The purpose of this book is to encourage you to cleanse yourself. This is not medical advice, nor a prescription, just good sense. You clean out your home, you clean out your car, and it is far more important and helpful to your well-being to clean out yourself.

The Clean-Me-Out Program

A method of self-healing and achieving
exceptional health Mother Nature's Way*
by
complete intestinal cleansing and
digestive rejuvenation

* God made Mother Nature

TABLE OF CONTENTS

1

INTRODUCTION

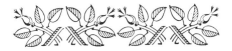

If an angel came and gave a formula that would cure almost any disease, it would be against the law to claim its effectiveness. But explaining in simple, scientific terms how we destroy our own bodies and minds and how we may reverse that destruction, leaving out all claims, will hopefully not offend the A.M.A. or F.D.A., will it? Fortunately, we live in a country that guarantees freedom of speech. Anyone is welcome to use a system of healing that has been proven to work, but they won't profit much monetarily. The health profession makes money on sick people, not well people. If we were to make everyone well with a system that works, we certainly wouldn't perpetuate our incomes. After all, there would be little use for this book, the "Clean-Me-Out Program," or even the entire health care system. How sincerely do we want to heal?

Evidence clearly states: no matter what the disease, as long as a person has the right mental attitude—in this case, a strong desire to be healthy and the willingness to do whatever is necessary to be cured—he will bring into his world that which he desires; he *will* find health. If only health professionals would espouse this truth, the door would open to making (or letting) it happen. Too often people lose hope because they continue to be treated by those whose healing successes are rare.

The Four Steps in Overcoming Disease

The **first** step in overcoming disease is to put a stop to its cause. This *always* begins with the re-arranging of the thoughts and feelings. For the decomposition of the body (or dying) *begins with* "suicidal" thoughts and feelings—i.e. feelings of hate, anger, criticism, condemnation, judgment, blame, self-pity, jealousy, resentment and depression. Good health requires not only the control of the emotions, but good thoughts and good feelings. Love, peace, harmony, poise, gratitude and praise expand the life and light in the body, building energy, vitality and happiness.

The **second** step toward perfect health of the body is to stop eating any foods that do not contain enzymes, life force and nutrients since lifeless "foods" cause mucus, toxins and congestion—especially congestion of the intestinal tract. This substance is known as "hardened mucoid fecal matter" and is the cause of over 90% of all disease (with the exception of injuries).

The **third** step toward overcoming disease is to remove congestion anywhere and everywhere from the body. Some health professionals choose to address the local area of obvious trouble alone. But, as Dr. Bernard Jensen likes to say, "if you step on a cat's tail, it's the other end that yells!" There is no single part of the body that is not affected by the whole. So, all congestion and toxins must be removed and it must begin with the removal of the hardened mucoid fecal matter.

The **fourth** step toward lasting health is to then supply the body with the needed elements. But you cannot successfully complete this step until the third step is done, or well on its way.

Nature's Own Remedy—A Logical Process

Isn't this sensible? This logical process is Nature's own remedy, yet it is in large part neglected by health professionals. This explains uncountable failures, for even when there is success in curing one ailment, it is rarely more than a brief time before the patient develops another ailment. This is because the symptom alone was treated, not the cause.

One prominent cancer researcher, Dr. Hardin Jones said, *"My studies have proved conclusively that untreated cancer victims actually live up to four times longer than treated individuals* . . . Beyond a shadow of a doubt, radical surgery on cancer patients does more harm than good." Dr. Jones said he advocates less surgery and chemotherapy. According to Edward Griffin, author of *World Without Cancer* (a fantastic book that I urge you to read), excluding skin cancer, the average cure rate of cancer by medical doctors is 17%. Would you take your car to a mechanic if he claimed a mere 17% cure rate of transmissions? I would suggest it is time to consider other methods.

The medical world claims no cure for cancer and, what's more, no one else can either. It's against the law—even for those who know the cure. Therefore, *I hereby announce that I do not claim the "Clean-Me-Out Program" will cure cancer.* Should you find your cancer disappearing when you use this system, I will not accept responsibility. You'll have to credit yourself.

The cure of cancer or any other disease *has been known for decades* among health experts who understand disease and its cause. But, it is also unlawful for those experts to treat cancer unless they are M.D.'s. What a crime against the American people! To think that there are those who can cure cancer who are not legally permitted to do it!

I had better be careful here. I had better not say that all cancers can be cured. No disease is curable if it's gone too far or if the patient's attitude will not permit healing. But based on the patients I've known who have conquered cancer, heart disease, diabetes and leukemia, based on the numerous books I've read and health professionals I've talked to, the following is undeniably true: America must look to other healing methods if it wants to return to the healthy nation it once was. There are some shocking governmental statistics to support this statement.

The Facts

The U.S. Public Health Service revealed the rate of health deterioration of the American people. Out of 100 participating nations of the world, America *was* the healthiest in 1900. In 1920, we dropped to the second highest nation. During World War II, we went back to number one—that's when sugar and meat were hard to get and family vegetable gardens were common. In 1978, we dropped to 79th. In 1980, we were *95th*! (I recently heard from a friend in the business of enlightened healing that we have now hit rock bottom—that's number *100* on the list.) Yet we are said to be the wealthiest nation in the world. *Who*, or *what*, is responsible?

A Departure from Nature

Since 1900, the basic, sensible theories of health care have changed dramatically. The major change was the shift from Nature, or natural healing methods, to drugs. In addition to this shift in health care came the increasing use of preservatives and chemicals taken into our bodies through food, polluted air and synthetic fabrics. This unnatural approach to life has had its detrimental effect on the American people.

In my opinion, as long as our approach to healing (except in rare cases) involves the use of drugs, chemicals, radiation and scapels, we will never be successful. If we sincerely want to bring the American people back to health, or if we personally wish to reclaim our own perfect health, we must return to God and follow His ways—Nature's ways—by using herbs and other natural methods that purify and strengthen the body.

How the "Clean-Me-Out Program" Developed

I started colon cleansing with a very popular program that claims "no cleansing reactions". After a month of feeling sluggish and rather depressed and not noticing a single positive result, I dropped it like a hot potato. I began researching and using other seven-day herbal colon cleansing programs and got what I then thought were great results - an average of 13 feet of hard, mucoid fecal substance came out of me that I can assure you wasn't just your average fecal excretions! Then Dr. Bernard Jensen convinced me to try pancreatin, which resulted in the elimination of 28 feet in seven days. However, pancreatin is an animal product, and I was determined to find something as effective without putting dead animal vibration in my body.

The next summer, I scheduled a research and experimenting expedition with an old friend of mine - White Medicine Crow - the most unusual herbalist I've ever known and as wild (maybe wilder) in the mountains as I am. We were to live off the land, eating fresh herbs only, live in the open air, take cold baths and study the human body. We started in Arizona. That was rough. Then the Mount Lassen area in California. That was heavenly. Then the Redwoods, the ocean, and it was about then that we began eliminating the famous "hardened mucoid fecal substance". And all without doing any so-called cleansing! This substance was coming not only from the colon, but from all areas of the intestines - even the duodenum. But which herbs were doing this? We had eaten so many! By the time we finished our research in the north Cascades, we knew which herbs produced the desired effect and put together a formula which has never been equalled. We tried it on ourselves. First time - *40 feet of mucoid fecal elimination in six days* for me and 28 feet for White Crow on his first cleanse ever. Talk about feeling good after that - WOW!

2

HOW PEOPLE MAKE THEMSELVES AND THEIR CHILDREN SICK

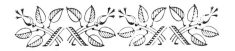

In a nutshell, people get sick because of negative thoughts and feelings, poor food combinations, chemicals and the wrong food. All of these things create congestion and toxins in the body.

Eating Devitalized Foods

Our bodies are designed to partake of raw foods only. Foods that have been cooked, frozen, canned or processed are dead foods, or actually no foods at all. Now I realize that the average American has not reached the point where he will accept or understand what I say, but I will say it anyway: the true definition of a food is "a substance that nourishes or fuels the body with life-giving force (i.e. vitamins, minerals, enzymes, etc.), thereby strengthening, energizing and building it." Food is not simply something one puts in the mouth, chews and swallows. Food should not deplete or rob the body of its needed essence or harm it in any way. Dead or dying foods take an enormous toll on the body. Consider these facts about cooked, frozen, canned and processed foods:

- they have been depleted of many vitamins
- they create toxins
- they drain the life force from the body

- they destroy the constructive bacteria in the intestines
- they poison the bloodstream, thereby feeding disease
- they clog the body's lymph system
- they drain the body's enzyme reserve
- they overwork and clog the elimination systems
- they strain the glandular system
- they overwork the digestive system
- they cause stress, congestion and mucus
- they produce the ideal environment for parasites

The Creation of Mucoid Substance

In addition to devitalized (decaying) foods, highly toxic substances such as coffee, candy, alcohol, spoiled food, and drugs (medicinal and otherwise) taken orally stimulate the body to automatically secrete a mucus substance throughout the alimentary canal. This is a natural, protective mechanism to prevent the absorption of toxins. Eating substance such as meat, or anything in a state of serious rot, triggers the protective mucus. I'm sure this protective mechanism was designed for the occasional mistake—like the time I drank some rotten orange juice. After the occasional mistake has triggered the body's protective mucoid layer, the pancreatic juices could easily strip it off within a few days.

However, most people have a habit of eating toxic substances with every meal and often in-between. The layers then become so thick that the pancreas' rescue mission is totally suppressed.

As we continue to eat toxic-producing substances, layer upon layer of mucoid matter builds in the entire alimentary canal, causing gradual weakening of the body. As these mucoid layers build up, the peristaltic action in the intestines becomes less and less effective. This is where problems really begin. As the peristalsis becomes more and more inhibited, transit time of food through the alimentary canal become slower and slower. As it slows, food begins to rot before it exits and also loses its moisture, causing it to become smelly, dry and sticky. It then has a tendency to stick to the walls of the intestines creating thicker and thicker layers of substance. Then it bulges and causes protrusions which can become diverticulitis, colitis and other colon problems, including colon cancer. All of this substance is extremely toxic and a major source of poisons or "free radicals" (the new terminology for toxins and poisons). Though this is a serious condition, the body works overtime to try and handle the toxic overloads. Yet, if this substance is not removed, the body fights a losing battle and eventually the immune system will break down, the liver, kidneys and skin will become clogged and tired, the enzymes will run low and the body will begin to deteriorate. And, as the decades go by, each generation becomes weaker, according to the hereditary constitution, strength of the digestive system, physical and mental activities and diet.

Ignoring the Intestinal Tract

In the early 1900's, Dr. J.H. Tilden of Denver, Colorado specialized in healing pneumonia, which was then the number one killer. He had more pneumonia cases than any other doctor and he never lost a patient. He used no drugs at all. He simply cleaned out the colon, used water therapy and administered natural, live foods. Even in those days his success was considered phenomenal because other doctors were relying on drugs and continually meeting with failure. It is estimated that over 90% of disease in America is attributable directly or indirectly to an unhealthy digestive tract. As Dr. Bernard Jensen puts it: *"Every tissue is fed by the blood, which is supplied by the bowel. When the bowel is dirty, the blood is dirty, and so on to the organs and tissues . . . it is the bowel that invariably has to be cared for first before any effective healing can take place."*

Dr. Jensen knows what he is talking about. (He has had one of the most successful careers in healing people in the 20th century. I believe he'll go down in history as one of the most effective pioneers in the health field.) Most Americans have serious problems in their intestinal tracts, whether they know it or not. People are unknowingly suffering from serious *malnutrition* (no matter what they eat, since their bodies can absorb so little) and *autointoxication* (self-poisoning) because of an accumulation of hardened mucoid fecal substance in the intestinal tract.

This accumulated substance may be several inches thick and go from the stomach through the entire length of both the small and large intestines. It's peculiar—the small intestine is called small, when it's actually six times longer than the large intestine, or colon. The small intestine is over 22 feet long and is of greater importance when considering malnutrition because mucoid substance in that area blocks assimilation of nutrients as well as reflex points (see the **Chart on Reflex Points**). Even those health care professionals who are enlightened as to the benefits of internal cleansing generally consider only the 4 - 6 feet of the colon. However, the *entire* intestinal tract and stomach must be cleansed of this mucoid substance.

Often layered, the mucoid substance can be so hard that it is difficult to cut with a knife. One autopsy revealed a colon nine inches in diameter, packed with layer upon layer of encrusted mucoid fecal material, leaving a tiny one-fourth inch opening. What's your waist line? If it's larger than you know it should be, keep reading. Another autopsy exposed a colon so packed with mucoid substance that it weighed 40 pounds! That's astounding, when you stop to consider that the healthy colon should weigh three to five pounds. This increased weight of the transverse colon weakens its structure and causes prolapsus, which in turn puts pressure upon the lower organs and weakens them (creating prostate, bladder and female problems).

During a cleanse, this old mucoid matter usually comes out in sections of one to two feet (the longest single piece known is 27 feet) and is generally thick, hard, stiff, green to black and sometimes very foul in odor. You may find worms as long as 5 - 20 feet come out, or yellow popcorn-looking substance, or (as excess lymph comes out) an amber or dark green jelly-like goop. Fun stuff! This is where cleansing becomes entertaining and educational. You will soon consider yourself a qualified "intestinal discharge" examiner. I keep a pair of chopsticks by my toilet during a cleanse for examination and ease in measuring. If several family members or friends cleanse at the same time, it's fun to keep track of the number of feet you get out and compare notes. No kidding! It's at least ten times more entertaining that the average TV sitcom and enormously more valuable.

11

Looking in the toilet and seeing that substance you will be filled with great joy, for you will be flushing away the cause of lack of energy, premature old age, failing eyesight, poor memory and most every disease. Loaded with drugs (which generally cannot be assimilated and are, therefore, stored in the body tissue), parasites and dead tissue, these old toxic substances, or free radicals, may flow from any and all channels of elimination during the cleanse— the kidneys, skin, lungs, mouth, nose and ears.

The Manufacturing of Free Radicals

When the intestines have any of this hardened mucoid substance there is an interference with the digestive process. Even if a person had just a thin layer of this substance lining the intestinal tract, he would have sluggish peristaltic action. As previously mentioned, this person would be suffering from some degree of malnutrition because food has difficulty being absorbed through a mucoid layer.

Any mucoid fecal build-up results in fermentation, putrifaction (rotting) and stagnant pus pockets holding various poisons and harmful bacteria (a state of autointoxication). This substance has its own low vibration and constantly radiates death into the mental and emotional bodies, further perpetuating negative feelings, thoughts and habits. Sometimes pockets of pus and debris settle and accumulate to such a degree that the colon's circumference expands to four or more times its normal size. Is it any wonder most people have bulging lower abdomens?

Occasionally, smaller pockets start protruding beyond the colon wall, forming diverticulitis. These conditions are perfect for worms and parasites. It is in these areas that colon cancer develops. You didn't really think that cancer just came without a cause, did you?

These toxins, poisons or free radicals constantly seep into the bloodstream and lymph, settling in the weaker areas of the body. As these weak areas give way to the toxic overloads, disease develops. As one health expert put it, "the name of a disease depends upon where the poisons settle. Thus, from the same source, various names of disease are given." Even if one succeeds in strengthening the weak area or suppressing the symptom, the toxic flow from the bowel will find another area to break through. *Disease can only permanently be overcome when the cause is remedied.*

If you can understand the last three paragraphs, you will know more about the cause of disease and its proper treatment than the medical world does. For if the medical world would try to understand this and treat the cause of disease with Nature's perfect methods designed for man by God, instead of relying on drugs, radiation and scapels designed by man, their continual failures would become successes. Though this would not enhance their pocketbooks, the planet would become a world of healthy people.

I was talking about treating causes with a fellow once who insisted, "When I get a flat tire I just fix it. I don't worry about causes." I replied, "Would you try to fix the leaking hole in the tire while the nail was still in it?" He said, "Oh. I see what you mean." Doctors do the very same thing when they cut out cancer in a colon or breast. They leave the cause. Patients go home and pray that it doesn't come back again. Seldom are they told to change their diets. They are rarely given nutritional advice. They go home and keep doing what they like to do—they are told to "enjoy life" if they can.

You may be wondering about radiation therapy—will that remove the cause? Emphatically no! After such severe treatments the whole body's immune system is essentially destroyed, since radiation destroys enzymes. The body is then so weak, how could it possibly go about healing itself? Such treatments are never the part of wisdom.

The Manifestations of Negative Energy

Although this book deals primarily with the physical body, the real cause of disease is negative thoughts and feelings. We live in a universe that is ruled by exact Law. Being ignorant of it does not does not mean we can in any way avoid its effect. As sound in its own octave is solid enough to impress itself upon our ear drums to hear, so are thoughts and feelings (in their own octave) real and solid. And they do not dissipate after they are created. Thoughts and feelings solidify not only into our worlds as conditions or things, but also solidify into our bodies and minds.

Mind is the Master Power
that molds and makes.

And man is mind
and forevermore he takes

his tools of thought
and shaping what he wills—

brings forth a thousand joys,
a thousand ills.

He thinks in secret,
and it comes to pass.

Environment
is but his looking glass.

(author unknown)

Consider the words of the Master Jesus: "Ye shall pay even the last penny." "That which you sow shall you also reap." "According to your faith it is done unto you." Most of us are affected by the past more than the Now. Thoughts and feelings of the past constantly seep into our brains, bodies and environments, producing the cause behind the cause. Man may be unjust, but Nature (God) is not. If we are not satisfied with our minds, bodies and conditions in our worlds as they are, we must "cleanse and purify" and "sin no more." I quote from *The Gospel of Peace of Jesus Christ* by the disciple John:

"I tell you in very truth, Man is the Son of the Earthly Mother, and from her did the Son of Man receive his whole body, even as the body of the newborn babe is born of the womb of his mother. I tell you truly, you are one with the Earthly Mother; she is in you, and you in her. Of her were you born, in her do you live, and to her shall you return again. Keep, therefore, her laws, for none can live long, neither be happy, but he who honors his Earthly Mother and does her laws. For your breath is her breath; your blood is her blood; your bone her bone; your flesh her flesh; your bowels her bowels; your eyes and your ears are her eyes and her ears.

"I tell you truly, should you fail to keep but one only of all

14

these laws, should you harm, but one only of all your body's members, you shall be utterly lost in your grievous sickness, and there shall be weeping and gnashing of teeth. I tell you, unless you follow the laws of your Mother, *you can in no wise escape death*. And he who clings to the laws of his Mother, to him shall his Mother cling also. She shall heal all his plagues, and he shall never become sick. She gives him long life, and protects him from all afflictions; from fire, from water, from the bite of venomous serpents. For your Mother bore you, keeps life within you. She has given you her body, and none but she heals you. Happy is he who loves his Mother and lies quietly in her bosom. For your Mother loves you, even when you turn away from her. And how much more shall she love you, if you turn to her again? I tell you truly, very great is her love, greater than the greatest of mountains, deeper than the deepest seas. And those who love their Mother, she never deserts them. As the hen protects her chickens, as the lioness her cubs, as the mother her newborn babe, so does the Earthly Mother protect the Son of Man from all danger and from all evils.

"For I tell you truly, evils and dangers innumerable lie in wait for the Sons of Men. Beelzebub, the prince of all devils, the source of every evil, lies in wait in the body of all the Sons of Men. He is death, the lord of every plague, and taking upon him *a pleasing raiment*, he tempts and entices the Sons of Men. Riches does he promise, and power, and splendid palaces, and garments of gold and silver, and a multitude of servants, all these; he promises renown and glory, fornication and lustfulness, gluttony and wine-bibbing, riotous living, and slothfulness and idle days. And *he entices every one by that to which their heart is most inclined.* And in the day that the Sons of Men have already become the slaves of all these vanities and abominations, then in payment thereof he snatches from the Sons of Men all those things which the Earthly Mother gave them so abundantly. He takes from them their breath, their blood, their bone, their flesh, their bowels, their eyes and their ears. And the breath of the Son of Man becomes short and stifled, full of pain and evil-smelling, like the breath of unclean beasts. And his blood becomes thick and evil-smelling, like the

15

water of the swamps; it clots and blackens, like the night of death. And his bone becomes hard and knotted; it melts away within and breaks asunder, as a stone falling down upon a rock. And his flesh waxes fat and watery; it rots and putrefies, with scabs and boils that are an abomination. *And his bowels become full with abominable filthiness, with oozing streams of decay; and multitudes of abominable worms have their habitation there.* And his eyes grow dim, till dark night enshrouds them, and his ears become stopped, like the silence of the grave. And last of all shall the erring Son of Man lose life. For he kept not the laws of his Mother, and added sin to sin. There, are taken from him all the gifts of the Earthly Mother: breath, blood, bone, flesh, bowels, eyes and ears, and after all else, life, with which the Earthly Mother crowned his body.

"But if the erring Son of Man be sorry for his sins and undo them, and return again to his Earthly Mother; and if he do his Earthly Mother's laws and free himself from Satan's clutches, resisting his temptations, then does the Earthly Mother receive again her erring Son with love and sends him her angels that they may serve him. I tell you truly, when the Son of Man resists the Satan that dwells in him and does not his will, in the same hour are found the Mother's angels there, that they may serve him with all their power and free utterly the Son of Man from the power of Satan.

"For no man can serve two masters. For either he serves Beelzebub and his devils or else he serves our Earthly Mother and her angels. *Either he serves death or he serves life.* I tell you truly, happy are those that do the laws of life and wander not upon the paths of death. For in them the forces of life wax strong and they escape the plagues of death."

Our bodies are supposed to be the temples of the Living God. Instead they have become seething, smelly cesspools that house fermenting, putrifying, rotting death. There are two main causes - that which we have eaten and the negatively-charged energy in the mental and feeling worlds which *physically* solidifies in the cell structure causing various malfunctions in the body.

You will prove this to yourself as you cleanse. For the deeper you cleanse the mucoid substance from your body, the more memories, thoughts, feelings, desires, tastes and smells from the past come to your consciousness. Some remembrances will come back very vividly even though you had totally forgotten them.

Most Americans have substance in their intestines that has been there since they were children—in some cases, babies. As this old substance breaks up, you may recall incidents that occurred when you ate the substance that is now coming out. Many temporarily feel the emotions they were feeling then when they ate something years ago. As long as the substance containing these emotions, thoughts or desires are still within you, you will be influenced by them. Hence, neurotic people fight a tough battle if they never cleanse. But once the mucoid substance containing those elements goes down the drain—presto!—you will not be influenced by it again.

The Problem With Eating Meat

You can now understand why the great spiritual geniuses of antiquity always fasted—often for 40 days or so before they achieved their exalted consciousness. As long as the negative consciousness is within, a heavy weight holds you low. Herein is the key to why no great spiritual genius would eat meat—for the negative feelings of fear, hate and death vibrate throughout the animal as it is being murdered. Who would want to digest that?

It took one year after I quit eating meat and several fasts before I rid myself of disturbed, low-vibratory feelings and the seeming inability to find peace within. This should make it obvious why we should *never eat when* the feeling world is stirred negatively. Refuse to do so from here on out! If you're still a meat eater and think you are happy, give up meat-eating for a year-and-a-half, cleanse or fast a few times and you will find a peace and happiness you never knew existed.

Parasites

Parasites and worms thrive in mucoid layers. They feed on it. They are protected from most vermifuges (de-worming measures) by burying themselves inside the impacted layers. There they remain, happily nestled in their perfect habitat, until the mucoid fecal layers are removed once and for all. Years ago I had suspected that I might have a tapeworm and who knew what else. After much cleansing of my intestinal tract I tried several herbal formulas to kill and extract the little buggers using black walnut, an herbal pumpkin formula, garlic and pumpkin seeds. I went on several weeks, off two weeks, and back on again to get the eggs. Later, Dr. Jensen told us that the only truly effective means he knew of to kill worms was to eat nothing but raw onions and garlic for three days and take a strong herbal laxative (overdose) the last night. The next morning we were to sit in warm milk when it was time for a movement. (As strange as this sounds, worms love warm milk. The theory is that the weakened worms will end up in the colon after fleeing from the raw onion and garlic, but scurry back up when feeling the cold air at the anus. If they sense the warm milk instead, they will go for it.)

Since my buddy White Crow and I never recommended anything we hadn't tried ourselves, we took off to the mountains. We went through three days of agony and even sat in the warm milk. The last part was the most hilarious moment of my life—but that shall remain confidential. The only thing that came out was a one-inch hookworm. About a year after my last major de-worming attempt, we were in Tucson. White Crow, my beloved wife and myself were all on the Cleanse but experimenting with eating one meal a day. At this time I felt I was about 90% cleaned out. About the only part of my digestive system that was not completely free of mucoid matter was the stomach. I was certain of this because I still had an apparent hydrochloric acid deficiency. We were on our fourth day of the Cleanse. I had just finished taking the psyllium shake (a part of the "Clean-Me-Out Program"). I suddenly gulped for air. I doubled over and grabbed by stomach. For about 20 minutes I had to hold my stomach and found that I couldn't stand up straight. I felt like something was trying to turn my stomach inside-out. It wasn't really painful, but was a very weird feeling. Then just as suddenly as it had come, it disappeared and never returned. The next morning I passed a worm about four feet long. And the morning after that I passed either another one or a piece of the previous one that was about a foot long. Once you start cleansing seriously, be aware that such an experience may happen to you. And be thankful.

Junk foods, and by that I mean any foods that are unnatural to a truly healthy body, overwork the stomach, pancreas, kidneys, liver, heart, thyroid and more. They severely strain the body's immune system. And they produce the ideal breeding ground for parasites.

Over 134 kinds of parasites can live in the human body. Most Americans have one kind or another. Parasite epidemics have occurred in New York, Colorado, Washington and New Hampshire, with serious outbreaks in other states. Parasites can even coat the inside lining of the small intestine and prevent the lining from absorbing nutrients in food. They can also cause severe constipation by blocking or plugging the alimentary canal. On a world-wide basis, worms outrank cancer as man's deadliest enemy. In fact, the World Health Organization has named parasitic diseases as among the six most harmful infective diseases in humans.

In Brazil one parasite called American Trypanosomiasis causes 30% of adult deaths. Relative to other countries, it was thought that North Americans suffered little from parasite diseases because of our "good health," "good nutrition," climate and sanitation. Climate, yes. Sanitation, yes. But the fact that we are one of the sickest nations in the world would reflect poor nutrition. Increasingly poor eating habits are beginning to catch up with each new generation. Parasite diseases in America have increased significantly just in the last two decades. Few medical doctors understand the significance of this. Seldom do they look for parasites in their patients. And even if they suspected parasites, few would know what to look for or how to *effectively* treat them.

I know of a doctor who was examining a patient's eyes with a microscope and saw a tiny worm crawl from one part of the eye to the other side and disappear. Parasites may be microscopic in size or as long as 20 feet (or longer). Most of them are not deadly, but they can cause a lot of trouble. Parasite disease symptoms mimic many other diseases, thereby avoiding accurate diagnosis.

Since the medical world does not accept the fact that parasites are abundant in the American people, they have not thoroughly investigated what parasite invasion can do throughout the body. Parasites can live anywhere in the body—be it intestines, lungs, liver, muscles or brain. One autopsy revealed five tapeworms in a woman's head. If they cause damage to the nerves in the head or spine, symptoms can occur anywhere in the body—from one end to the other. Similarly, if worms are in the intestinal tract, they can cause problems in the heart, liver, kidneys, brain, etc. by their toxic secretions or by reflex disturbance.

Here is a partial list of parasite disease symptoms. Do you ever have symptoms like these?

Dizziness	Rashes
Diarrhea	Shortness of breath
Malnutrition	B-12 deficiency
Abdominal pain	Weakness
Weight loss	Colitis
Weight gain	Irritability
Anorexia	Bloody spit
Burning urination	Headaches
Coughing	Bleeding rectum
Fevers	Chest pains
Itching	Vomiting
Night sweating	Chills
Nausea	Burping
Blood in feces	Anemia
Sweating	Weak immunity
Joint pain	Jaundice
Muscle pain/spasms	Skin ulcers
Rectal prolapsus	Blurry vision
Loss of sleep	Blindness

Digestive disturbance
Lung and bronchial congestion
Acute muscular inflammation
Disfigurement of various body parts
Typhoid fever symptoms
Acute, chronic constipation
Vaginal inflammation with yellow, frothy foul-
    smelling discharges
Central nervous system impairment

Swelling of eyes, face, etc.
Malaria-like chills and fevers
Enlargement and malfunction of organs such as liver,
    spleen, lymph nodes, heart, gall bladder, etc.

You may be asking how a clean-living person could possibly become infested with parasites. Some of the more serious infections (especially those involving large worms) find their way into the human body when one eats rarely-cooked pork, beef, fish or any other creatures that have eyeballs, legs, fins or pinchers (yes, that includes crab and lobster).

Touching dogs, cats and other animals may lead to one's picking up parasite eggs or sometimes parasites themselves. Here are other methods of infection:

- Drinking infected water
- Being bitten by flies, mosquitoes and animals
  (usually in the tropics)
- Contacting filthy environments through breathing
  or touching (remember, just like cockroaches,
  parasites thrive in a filthy environment)
- Eating foods grown in infected soil, especially soil
  which has been fertilized with animal dung (pig
  dung is particularly contagious)
- Eating unclean, raw vegetation (wash your vegetables!)
- Walking barefooted on infected soil

Some common worms such as roundworms lay over 200,000 eggs a day. Hookworms lay 5 - 10,000 eggs a day and can live for about fourteen *years*. Something to think about. Once parasites are in the body the only sure way to get them out is to get rid of their environment of filth. Take away their environment and they will go away with the help of herbal vermifuges. Remember the promise and take heart: *"Cleanse and purify thyself and I will exalt thee to the throne of power!"*

3

BENEFITS OF THE "CLEAN-ME-OUT PROGRAM"

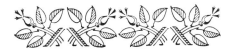

I have investigated most of the intestinal cleanses on the market, and by that I mean I have used them on myself. The "Clean-Me-Out Program" is, without a doubt, the easiest and most effective, powerful and complete intestinal cleansing program available.

Developing "Chomper"

The key to the Program's success is an herbal combination called *"Chomper Intestinal Reamer Cleaner"* which was developed almost by accident. After spending many years using other cleanses (usually just colon cleanses), I found several herbs that had a powerful effect in loosening and dissolving that horrible hardened mucoid plaque. By eating these herbs in their fresh state, mixed in what we called "wild salads" for a month or two, we joyously found the mucoid matter coming out with nearly every bowel movement. This was while eating two large salads daily.

Knowing what a valuable discovery this was, I was thrilled. I knew all too well how difficult it was to remove that slow death from the intestines. I knew how seriously the mucoid matter contributed to almost every disease known to man. I began to put together my herbal formula. I wanted the combination to be able to do the following:

- dissolve and break up mucoid matter
- rapidly expel mucoid matter from the system
- cause no cramping
- reduce gas in the stomach and intestines
- kill any possible infection and heal any sore areas
- purify the blood
- stimulate and strengthen all organs, especially the heart, liver and eliminative organs
- increase the secretions of the liver, pancreas and stomach
- strengthen, heal and re-build the peristaltic action as well as the entire digestive system
- take away appetite
- calm the nervous system and reduce possible pain
- kill some worms
- stop any hemorrhages which wouldn't likely occur anyway

In short, it had to act as an aperient, alterative, tonic, antispasmodic, antisphiletic, nervine, astringent, detergent and stomachic. I tried the combination I developed on myself and then on White Crow, who agreed that it would have no negative side effects as long as the correct proportions were used. But when we took extremely heavy doses we felt pressure and spaciness in the head. We knew that one of the herbs in the combination (plantain) was the cause because it removes mucus from the head. After making the necessary adjustments, we were ready for the Cleanse.

Fantastic Results

We were not to eat anything during the Cleanse. Six days later, having never experienced hunger, I had passed a total of 40 feet of unbelievably gnarly mucoid matter. White Crow had passed 28 feet—and this on his *first* cleanse, taking no enemas, and getting up in the night on the fourth day of cleansing and having a potato feast! Of course, this slowed him down. But he went around telling everyone how much he got out and how wonderful he felt.

I'll never forget the day we stopped at an herb shop in Seattle. White Crow struck up a conversation with the owner who had also designed his own cleanse. This fellow was totally convinced that his cleanse was the best in the country. White Crow began telling him about the "Clean-Me-Out Program" and when he mentioned passing 28 feet in seven days, I'll never forget that fellow's face! I walked over and told him about my 40 feet. His jaw dropped open. Then he turned and walked away without a word. Poor fellow—I suppose he figured we were a couple of liars!

My wife's first cleanse was just as successful. Having only done one other "cleanse" before and getting nothing out at all, she was only doing it to appease me. In seven days she passed 37 feet of the old, mucoid gunk and a few parasites. She was so thrilled she continued to cleanse about every seven weeks and intends to keep cleansing until nothing more comes out!

"Renew yourselves and fast. For I tell you truly, that Satan and his plagues may only be cast out by fasting and by prayer."
(Jesus—*The Gospel of Peace of Jesus Christ* by the Disciple John)

Testimonials

A lady in Rosemead, California wrote to us that she had gone from doctor to doctor and hospital to hospital because of a pain in her abdomen. She continues, "Before the end of the Cleanse, the pain was gone and I eliminated 50 feet. I was excited. I went another day and got eight more feet out!" She now holds the record and truly deserves a medal for her determination.

The glowing reports and happy testimonials continue to come in. Though I always expected the best, I admit to being amazed at the some of the letters. Seventy-eight-year-old Fred was so pleased with his results, he spread his 45 feet of "beautiful mucoid sheaths" (his own words) onto aluminum foil in the bathroom and took pictures!

One woman suffering from painful swelling in her neck and

"critical high blood pressure" said that after going to many doctors over the years without help for her problems, she went on the Cleanse for six days. The pain and swelling of her neck completely disappeared and her blood pressure returned to normal.

Another person said that his hemorrhoids were gone in seven days after the Cleanse. Letters and reports say that eyesight has improved, memory is better, and dry skin and wrinkles are diminishing after cleansing with the Program. Almost everyone reports a significant increase in energy and a general feeling of well-being after taking the Cleanse. Two people noticed that their gray hair is gradually disappearing as they cleanse with the Program. And several people have said that while on the Cleanse and, even after it, they feel closer to God. "Chomper" is being praised as a God-send, which it truly is. Mother Nature simply can't be improved upon. One checker at a health food store joked, "People are buying that *Chomper* like *M & M's!*" If only that were true.

Creating "Herbal Nutrition"

After I had experimented on myself and White Crow with success, I began to get serious about distributing this Cleanse to others. To make sure that their bodies would get all the protection and substance it required while cleansing, I always highly recommended they take a number of additional single herbs as I had always done. But this seemed costly and quite a bother. So I began to work on another formula which is now called *"Herbal Nutrition"* that would allow the maintenance of maximum strength, energy and optimal elimination from the appropriate organs. This combination, therefore, had to supply the body with the following:

- every vitamin and mineral in their perfect combinations
- digestive enzymes
- all trace minerals
- essential amino acids
- plenty of vitamin C, calcium, iron and potassium
- the correct balance of vitamin D, magnesium and

phosphorous which, in correct proportions along with the digestive enzymes, would assure assimilation of the calcium

- natural buffering agents for each ingredient
- stimulation to the lymph system
- plenty of B vitamins, vitamin A and zinc
- chlorophyll
- deodorizing effects (not essential, but a good idea)
- food (herbs) for the pituitary gland as well as whatever would assist "Chomper" in strengthening the heart, liver, kidneys, skin and the circulation

When "Herbal Nutrition" eventually came to the point where it satisfied all those requirements, I knew it was a fantastic product. Every vitamin and mineral supplement I knew of on the market seemed seriously out of balance with Nature. It therefore seemed clear that anyone who knew much about Nature, vitamins, minerals, buffering agents, drugs, the dissection of natural ingredients, combinations, digestion, assimilation and the meaning of organic vs. inorganic would be much happier with "Herbal Nutrition" than with what was generally found on the market.

Never Feel Hunger

No one ever believes us when we say that while on the Cleanse, you won't get hungry. At least, not until they have taken the Cleanse for the first time. You will be so full of herbs and juices that you just won't feel hungry. You may still struggle with the desire to eat, nonetheless, because of old, old habits.

For maximum cleansing, a full seven-day program with no food should be followed. Some people even like to go ten days. I wouldn't go any longer. Occasionally, there is the person who simply hasn't the self-control or determination to make it seven days without food, even though the body is getting every vitamin and mineral it needs from the herbs. For this reason, there are two approaches to the

"Clean-Me-Out Program." *Phase I - Go For It* is for the stronger individual who wants to be cleaned out fast. *Phase II - Easy Does It* is for the person who is not in such a hurry or who wants to cleanse cautiously. Both will get results, but Phase II will be considerably slower in dumping the toxic substance since it allows for the intake of some slightly steamed vegetables or fresh fruit once a day.

More Than One Cleanse?

The substance that can be removed during a seven-day period may astound you. And you should enjoy a noticeable improvement in your health within a few days after cleansing. I don't know a single exception to this. However, <u>seven days of cleansing will not remove all the encrusted mucoid layers</u> in the intestinal tract. Many, many years have been spent building layer upon layer of this substance throughout the entire alimentary canal. There is practically no limit as to how thick the layers can become. On a thin person the layers may be one-fourth of an inch thick. A heavy person tends to accumulate more. One colon was known to be 18 inches thick in diameter! Six to eight weeks after your first cleanse, another seven-day cleanse may be taken. (Note: If you are following the Phase II-Easy Does It you can cleanse much more often.) If this program is followed and nutritious eating habits are maintained, within two to three years, a state of health can be achieved that will amaze you. This has been found to be true of people even 80 years old. Again, this depends on:

- the condition you are presently in
- how closely you follow the Cleanse instructions
- how well you eat between cleanses
- which program you are following (Phase I or II)

Right now you may be thinking—I'm not even sure I want to do one cleanse, let alone one every six-to-eight weeks! To you, my friend, let me simply encourage you to try it for the first time. Even if you only did the Cleanse once a year, you would be giving your body enormous relief, saving it from the tiresome task of spending all its energy digesting and protecting itself from the overload of toxic matter we thoughtlessly dump into it three times a day (this doesn't even include snacking and coffee breaks). How much is your health worth to you? This once-a-year vacation would give the body a chance to take a breather and devote its energy to healing itself. And, besides, you may change your mind once you make it through the first time. The most important thing is to muster your courage and venture a first step into the unknown. It's true. It's not everyone who can do this. You will be distinguishing yourself from the lot of mankind who accepts ill-health as a cruel twist of fate and unconsciously struggles through life, accepting it blindly as it is. You will be proud of yourself and realize the stuff of which you are really made once you have completed your first cleanse.

Cleansing the Entire Gastrointestinal Tract

It should be noted that the "Clean-Me-Out Program" will cleanse the entire gastrointestinal tract or alimentary canal—all the way from the tip of the tongue to the anus. Although the colon tends to accumulate thicker layers than the other areas, the majority of what you will see coming out of you will be from the small intestine. The next two pages show drawings of various shapes and striations of the intestinal wall. After adhering to the side walls for so many years, the mucoid layers naturally take on the same shapes and creases. Studying these drawings you can identify the locality, or source, of your evacuations.

Sections of the Intestines

This can be very interesting. For example, if the substance came from the duodenum area (the small intestine next to the stomach), you know that the secretions from the pancreas, liver, and gall bladder ducts (the source of many digestive enzymes) have been blocked. Therefore, you can assume that your body's ability to digest

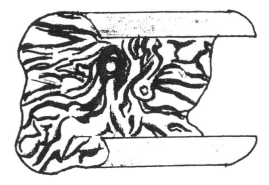

Figure A — Duodenum - located just below the stomach. About ten inches in length. Here important digestive juices from the gall bladder and pancreas enter the intestines. It is also in the duodenum where important digestive enzymatic activities should occur to prepare food for proper digestion. When it is covered with mucoid layers, the digestive juices remain under the layers and never reach the food. Note the direction of the striations or folds of the duodenum. Observe also the circles which represent the pancreatic and bile ducts.

Figure B — Jejunum - Located just below below duodenum. About eight-and-a-half feet long. Here the special cells of the intestinal wall secrete various chemicals to be combined with gall bladder and pancreatic juices. In this manner, the small intestine controls the digestive processes. The majority of nutrients are assimilated here and in the ileum. Note how the folds in the jejunum are large, closely packed and run in one direction.

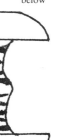

Figure C — Upper Ileum - Located just below the jejunum. About twelve feet in length with the lower ileum. Assimilation is its major function. Note that the folds are low and begin to fade away as it approaches the colon.

29

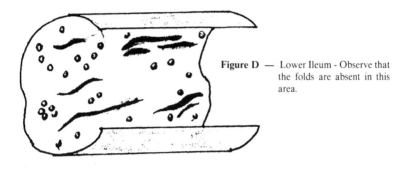

Figure D — Lower Ileum - Observe that the folds are absent in this area.

Figure E — Example of a mucoid particle from the colon - On your cleanse, you can expect to find mucoid substance shaped like this but much longer. When you see these, you know you are removing blockages to major lymph drainage areas.

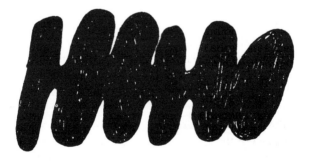

food properly has been greatly impaired. Hopefully, your first cleanse eliminated all obstructions in this area. If not on the first cleanse, maybe the next. But you see how important this could be. For if this area is covered with layers of mucoid fecal substance, the secretions from the digestive glands would just flow under the mucoid matter, never even reaching your food! If the mucoid layers exerted sufficient pressure, a back-up could occur in the glands, causing sluggish activity or even a possible shut-down of those glands. One doctor, after 50 years of service, claims over 85% of the population he dealt with had liver problems. This could be why. And this may give us hints about the possible causes of diabetes and hypoglycemia since both depend upon the proper functioning of the pancreas.

Most nourishment is assimilated in the small intestine (which is composed of the duodenum and upper and lower jejunum and ileum), although some nourishment may be absorbed through the stomach and colon. If you notice mucoid substance coming from the jejunum and ileum, you would again know that your body's ability to assimilate food properly has been greatly impaired. You could have been eating the most perfect, organic foods to no avail. Along with the presence of the mucoid layers is usually an imbalanced intestinal flora (with the presence of bacillus coli and other offensive coli bacteria). It is estimated that these toxic, undesirable organisms rule in 85% of the U.S. population (some say 95%). They produce sometimes bizarre reactions and consistently break down healthy tissue and drain a person's energy. They are also the main cause of gas.

Some of these coli bacteria have been known to cause cancer in laboratory animals. Most people who have cancer never find out why. It is interesting to note that cancer among meat eaters is *90% higher* than among life-long vegetarians. And the primary sustenance of the bacillus coli is meat. Next on the list of causes are overcooked foods and undigested proteins. Meat substitutes are high on the list as one of the primary detrimental foods for vegetarians. Once the body is cleansed of the causes of the imbalanced intestinal flora, it is imperative to replace the harmful bacteria with "friendly bacteria"–i.e. acidophilus, bifidus and streptococcus. This subject is thoroughly discussed in **Chapter 8 — "Eating for Good Health"** in the section entitled *"Healthy Bacteria"*.

Once the entire gastro-intestinal tract is cleansed of the hardened mucoid matter and you are consistently eating foods that maintain that purity, you will begin to reap the benefits. Actually, just getting a little out will help enormously.

Absorption of Nutrients

Now the body can absorb the nutrients from the food you eat. And you will be surprised at how little food it needs. Once "cleansed", a woman ate only one small meal every other day for two years. She reported that never had she felt so mentally alert. Never had she felt so good. So many people before cleansing absorb only a tiny portion of the nutrients in their food—no matter how nutritious the food and how much they eat. After thorough cleansing, there is no thick wall to prevent the absorption of nutrients.

Increased Peristaltic Action of the Intestines

The transit period of your food moving through the digestive tract is now shorter. As long as this continues, you will never be constipated again and you will not continue to build up mucoid fecal matter. The food, moving through more quickly, will no longer lose its moisture and become sticky and hard. This means you have removed the cause of the formation of pockets, bulges, diverticulitis, prolapsus and a host of other colon problems and disease.

Removal of the Source of Disease

Now you have eliminated the cause of putrification and fermentation; you have eliminated the perfect breeding environment for billions of diseased bacteria, germs and parasites. Therefore, the blood and every cell of your body is no longer being poisoned. Major organs are no longer being overloaded and working overtime, trying to correct and eliminate toxins. Now the body can rapidly repair the damage done in the past. And *the miracle of the body is that it will repair itself*; all it requires is the freedom from congestion and the proper nutrients to do it. When no longer spent on needed repairs, your energy can now flow to the mind or higher centers. Marvelous ideas, clear thinking, joy and love can now predominate.

Prolapsus Adjustment

Oftentimes the weight and pressure of many layers of hardened fecal matter, coupled with gravity over a period of time, have caused prolapsus of the transverse colon. The stomach may have dropped into what is called a "fishhook" position and cause further digestive problems with its over-acidity. As mentioned previously, the prolapsus also exerts pressure on the lower organs and is the main cause of bladder and urinary problems, various imbalances of the nerve centers, prostate ailments and most uterus and female problems. All of these conditions can repair themselves after the removal of the mucoid layers and by the use of certain herbs and exercises.

Improvement of Nerve Flow

It is well known that millions of nerves pass through the spinal column. When a vertebrae is out of place, a pinched nerve may develop, seriously affecting the area of that nerve attachment. Similarly, but not so dramatically, there are nerve reflex points in the intestines. When the intestinal tract is no longer plagued with fecal and mucoid impaction, the nerve supply is no longer in danger of short-circuiting, or developing a condition at the other end of the nerve.

Obliteration of Obesity

Many times overweight people will arrive at a point in cleansing when lymph drainage areas become unclogged and they drain "bucket loads" of lymph. These lucky people lose a good deal of "excess luggage."

The lymphatic system has many drainage areas—the most important of which is the colon. When it is impacted with mucoid layers, the lymphatic system gets blocked and back-up develops. This is one of the main reasons for obesity. When toxins cannot escape faster than they are being produced, the protective lymph wraps the toxic cells in its own liquid substance and stores them away.

The cleansing of the alimentary canal makes it possible to purify the lymphatic system, the blood, the brain and the entire body. You will enjoy greater health, energy, endurance, strength and mental alertness. *Expect to live a longer life,* looking and feeling good to the end, digesting and assimilating properly the smaller portions of food your body will now require! In fact, you may decide not to die at all and prefer to watch your body become younger instead of older. This is not a claim. But it is a goal for such a high level of attainment that the masses of mankind have not only lost all memory of it but, indeed, choose not at this time to accept it.

Shrinking the Abdomen

Mucoid layers eventually stretch the intestinal wall especially the colon. Those people boasting the famous "beer belly" and others whose stomachs fold over the belt, or those who cannot see their feet when they stand up straight can be sure that they have thick and dangerous mucoid build-up in the intestinal tract.

Once the mucoid layers are removed, the seriously-stretched intestines are still soft and flabby. But there is hope for a normal and healthy look—blessed herbs! After cleansing, white oak bark and ginger, when used properly, can draw the flesh back to its original position.

Take three capsules each of white oak bark and ginger root three times a day for about ten days. This will help tighten the cell tissue in the alimentary canal.

You can make a tea of equal parts white oak bark and ginger root. Just take some distilled water and lightly simmer pieces of these herbs for about ten minutes. You can use about one teaspoon of each herb per quart. More if you want it stronger, less if you like it weaker. It will not taste bad. If you use powdered herbs, place one half teaspoon of each herb in a cup and add boiling water and let it steep until cool enough to drink. Never drink anything too hot and never use aluminum pots to cook in or heat water.

For those with prolapses of the transverse colon, use the herbs as mentioned above, and also use a slant board. Lie on the slant board with the head down, and with your hands gently massage the abdomen, especially the transverse colon, in the direction of your head. Just reach as deep as you can and draw your intestinal tubes up. Visualize them staying in place. Remember, your mind is the controlling factor in your life. Whatever you accept as true will become a reality.

The Iris of the Eye

On page 36 is a chart on the iris of the eye which was developed by Dr. Bernard Jensen. Each point of the iris reveals the condition of its corresponding part of the body. It reflects the various stages of degeneration and conditions of the cell tissue. After you cleanse, note the changes in your iris. The changes in your body will usually take about three weeks to be reflected in the iris.

CHART TO IRIDOLOGY

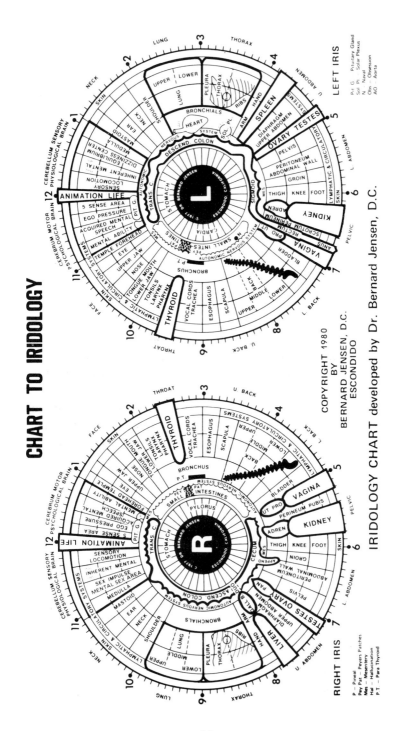

IRIDOLOGY CHART developed by Dr. Bernard Jensen, D.C.

COPYRIGHT 1980
BY
BERNARD JENSEN, D.C.
ESCONDIDO

LEFT IRIS

Pit G Pituitary Gland
Sol Pl Solar Plexus
N Naval
Obs. — Obsession
AO — Aorta

RIGHT IRIS

P — Pineal
Pey Pat — Peyers Patches
Mes — Mesentery
Hal — Hallucination
P T — Para Thyroid

36

4

HOW TO DETERMINE IF YOU NEED THE CLEANSE

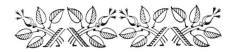

'' 'The message well I hear, but faith, alas is wanting.' Yes, the faith in a helper and savior is often put to a hard test here. The sick have been deceived so often and have buried all hope.''   (Adolf Just)

If you've been living on raw fruits and vegetables all your life, chances are you don't need the Cleanse. However, if you have any of the following you are most likely in serious need of intestinal cleansing:

- any disease or malfunction of the body
- constipation
- bad breath
- body odor
- flatulence (gas)
- dry and hard stools (they should be soft and break up when you flush the toilet)
- stools that sink (they should float)
- foul-smelling stools (they should not have bad odor and should be light brown; elimination of past meals should occur within 30 minutes after even a light meal—this may not happen until the intestinal

tract is completely cleansed, the peristaltic activity
rebuilt with herbs and the intestinal flora of both
the small and large intestines restored)

• evacuations that take more than 30 seconds or require
pushing or grunting (it should be quick and easy)

• tiny dark spots on the iris, about 1/5 of the distance
from the pupil to the outer circumference of the
iris, where there is usually a clear demarcation line
on the circle which surrounds the pupil; this circle
marks the digestive tract; these spots indicate either
diverticulitis or serious bowel pockets of long-
lasting congestion; the darker they are, the longer
they have been there and the more serious the
condition; if there are dark lines or spokes (radii
solaris) running from this area toward the
circumference, there are very likely parasites, too; if
this area is either lighter or darker than the rest of
the iris, there is some digestive disorder; refer to
the **Chart on Iridology** and note the area from the
pupil to the autonomic nervous system; this is the
area we are talking about.

Other ways to know if you need the Cleanse are: if you've ever
taken antibiotics (they completely destroy the friendly intestinal
flora), if you do not feel good, and if you lack energy. The diagram
on the next page is a chart of the colon and its reflex points. When
bowel pockets accumulate, you will generally have problems in the
areas indicated at the various reflex points. *Do you have any soreness
in the colon area?* Check the reflex points on this chart. If you have
problems in the areas indicated, you now know the cause. And you
can be sure that cleansing the colon (as well as the entire intestinal
tract) will be one of the best ways to get rid of those problems.

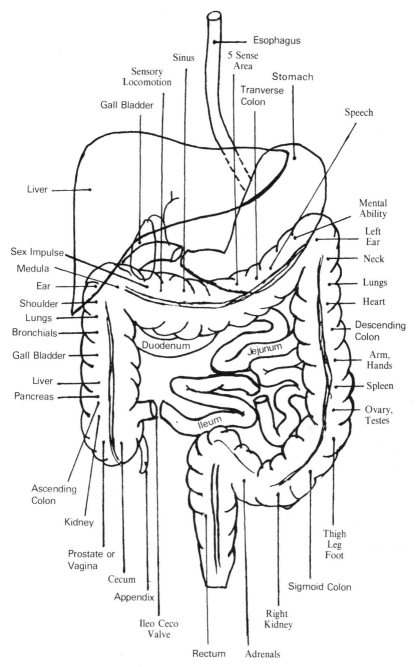

Reflex Points of the Colon

39

5

INGREDIENTS OF THE "CLEAN-ME-OUT PROGRAM"

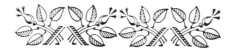

"CHOMPER INTESTINAL REAMER CLEANER" consists of plantain, barberry bark, myrrh, rhubarb root, fennel seed, ginger root, cascara sagrada bark, golden seal, capsicum, red raspberry leaf and lobelia. The following is a brief description of the benefits of these wonderful herbs:

PLANTAIN is one of the greatest herbs for breaking up the intestinal mucoid substance. It is one of the best blood purifiers known. A good liver herb, plantain also works well to improve the functioning of the kidneys. It helps to prevent gas and diarrhea. Overall, it is one of Nature's greatest healing herbs. Delicious in a salad (along with leaves of dandelion), you'll probably find it growing in your own backyard!

BARBERRY BARK is a powerful stomach and intestinal cleanser as well as a blood purifier. It helps to eliminate constipation and mucoid substance. Containing important antiseptic properties, barberry bark helps all liver problems.

MYRRH helps build the immune system and is one of the most effective stomach and intestinal cleansers/healers around. A wonderful antiseptic herb, myrrh helps rebuild the digestive system and remove gas.

RHUBARB ROOT acts as a tonic to the liver and gall ducts.

Although a laxitive, it checks diarrhea. It cleanses the mucous membranes in the digestive system and helps remove mucoid build-ups. Rhubarb is a major intestinal and liver cleanser. High in A and B complex and calcium, it helps rebuild the digestive system, reduce blood pressure and inflammation.

FENNEL SEED helps take away appetite. It helps remove waste from all parts of the body. It improves digestion and removes gas as well as killing pinworms and calming the nervous system.

GINGER ROOT removes congestion, relieves headaches and other aches and pains and is an effective bowel cleanser. Ginger improves the effect of the other herbs in "Chomper". It also improves circulation, settles the stomach and reduces fever and gas.

CASCARA SAGRADA BARK keeps things moving and rebuilds the peristaltic action in the intestines. It stimulates the gall bladder and adrenal glands. It has a major effect in removing the mucoid substance and in rebuilding the digestive system by increasing the secretions of the stomach, liver and pancreas.

GOLDEN SEAL stops infections and eliminates poisons. A blood purifier, aperient and alternative for mucous membranes, it helps to regulate liver functions and remove mucus from the nasal areas, bronchials, throat, intestines, stomach and bladder.

CAPSICUM is one of the most valuable herbs in the medical world. It is absolutely harmless, yet it is the most powerful stimulant known. Nothing can stop heart attacks or strokes faster, safer or more effectively than capsicum. It brings power and strength to the body. It heals stomach and intestinal ulcers. Nothing stops bleeding as well as capsicum. This marvelous herb greatly assists the cleansing and rebuilding of the digestive system and increases the effectiveness of other herbs. I could sing it praises forever, but I think you get the idea. (Included only in Original Formula)

RED RASPBERRY LEAF helps prevent hemorrhages and diarrhea. Supplying iron to the system, it helps build blood and increases energy. It also creates an astringent and contracting activity within the intestinal membranes that helps dislodge mucoid crust, eliminate constipation and other intestinal problems while improving digestion.

LOBELIA removes congestion and other obstructions from the body. It is an excellent herb for the elimination channels, especially lymph.

It is a great help in cases of cramps or pain. Dr. Thompson (a famous herbalist) said there is no herb more powerful than lobelia in the prevention and removal of disease. Many use it to induce vomiting. It is known to help remove catarrh, spasms, worms, fever, lung problems and nervousness. Another precious gift from Nature!

"HERBAL NUTRITION" consists of alfalfa, watercress, suma, dandelion, shavegrass (horsetail), irish moss, hawthorn berry, kelp, licorice root, rose hips and yellow dock. More on the virtues of these herbs follows:

ALFALFA is so high in vitamins and minerals that it is actually easier to list what it doesn't have. It lacks only vitamin B1, P and T. It has everything else! Alfalfa is noteworthy for its exceptional amount of trace minerals, for having all eight essential digestive enzymes, all eight essential amino acids and for being so high in vitamin A, K, and D, calcium, phosphorus, iron and potassium. It increases energy and endurance and helps digestion and the assimilation of calcium, protein and other nutrients. A body cleanser, natural deoderizer, builder and infection fighter, alfalfa contains chlorophyll. It is said to neutralize cancer.

WATERCRESS is one of the most nutritious foods known, was one of the main herbs in our meadow diet which produced the wondrous effect of eliminating undesirable mucoid plaque. It is a purifying herb that helps to eliminate all types of accumulations (cysts, tumors, stones, polyps, etc.) and their related diseases, such as: rheumatism, arthritis, and liver and kidney diseases.

SUMA (Pfaffia Paniculata) is an herb similar to ginseng. It is especially effective in strengthening the immune system, as it supplies the body with nutrients that build natural energy reserves. Perhaps this is why Suma has proven to be one of the most powerful herbs for the elimination of cancer.

DANDELION is one of the richest sources of vitamins and minerals in the herb kingdom. It is high in vitamin A, C, E and the B vitamins, potassium, calcium and organic sodium. A blood purifier, dandelion helps anemia. It also cleanses and stimulates the liver and helps hypoglycemia, rheumatism and gall bladder, spleen and stomach problems.

SHAVEGRASS (Horsetail) is high in silica which helps the body assimilate calcium. It is rich in selenium, pantothenic acid, paba, copper, manganese, cobalt, iron and iodine. It contains vitamin E. Shavegrass is good for circulation, the bladder, glands, kidneys, liver, hair and fingernails.

IRISH MOSS has an exceptionally high content of nutrients. It supplies vitamin A, D, E, F and K and is high in iodine (one mineral not found in most diets), calcium and sodium. (Note: the number one cause of arthritis is the lack of organic sodium and an excess of inorganic sodium.) Irish moss also contains phosphorous, potassium, organic sulphur, plus 15 of the 18 elements composing the body. It's good for the bladder, intestines and glands (especially thyroid). It aids bronchitis, cancer, goiter, tumors, varicose veins and lung and joint ailments.

HAWTHORN BERRY has been used for centuries in treating heart disease; it prevents arteriosclerosis and helps strengthen heart muscles. It is good for the heart valves and fast, weak or enlarged hearts. Good for angina pectoris and difficult breathing caused by ineffective heart activity and lack of oxygen, hawthorn berry is an antiseptic and good for the kidneys. It helps high and low blood pressure, rheumatism, hypoglycemia and arthritis.

KELP is a rich source of vitamin A, B1, B2, B3, B6, B12 (and every other B complex), C, E, G, K and S. Kelp contains at least 28 minerals, including every trace mineral. Containing, in addition, large amounts of iodine, it is able to feed the glandular system and help digest food by assisting the thyroid and other glands that affect digestion and by stimulating the digestive secretions of the stomach and pancreas. Kelp feeds the pituitary, thus affecting the entire body. It stimulates metabolism and helps burn up excess calories. It helps remove plaque from the arteries, gall bladder and kidneys. Very good for the complexion, wrinkles and skin, kelp cleanses and strengthens the entire body. It's a good herb for asthma, diabetes, eczema and goiter.

LICORICE ROOT is primarily in this combination because it helps balance the other herbs chemically (assiting pH levels). It gives a better flavor to the formula, which some people use in fruit smoothies and on their food as a seasoning. Giving energy and endurance to the system, licorice root contains vitamin E, B-complex, lecithin, manganese and zinc. Good for hypoglycemia and the removal of age spots and drugs from the body, it is also known to improve circulation and cleanse the blood, bronchials, throat and lungs.

ROSE HIPS is very rich in the B-complexes as well as vitamin A, E, C and rutin. It also contains vitamin D and P. Very good for the skin, rose hips is high in iron, calcium, potassium and silica. It helps stop infections, dizziness, cramps, colds, cancer, psoriasis and stress. It is also known to be a blood purifier.

YELLOW DOCK is 40% iron, which is the main reason it was included in "Herbal Nutrition." The best overall tonic for the entire system, it is used to treat anemia, cancer, leprosy and leukemia. A good liver and spleen herb, yellow dock is a major blood purifier and builder that also stimulates the elimination channels (especially the skin) and promotes the elimination of excess lymph.

Other Items Needed for the Cleanse

LIQUID BENTONITE acts like a magnet or sponge, absorbing toxic debris from the entire alimentary tract. It can absorb 180 times or more its own weight in toxins, bacteria and parasites. It should be used with psyllium husk powder. Then it pulls the loosened mucoid layers from the walls of the intestinal tract. The loosened matter then adheres to the bulk of the psyllium, allowing a quick exit in large pieces from the body.

PSYLLIUM HUSK POWDER swells when used with liquid bentonite and other liquids, producing a mass of soft jelly-like substance. It takes on the shape of the intestinal canal, acting like a broom and sweeping clean any loosened substance. In cooperation with "Chomper," this is a very important part of the Program.

CHLOROPHYLL is exceptionally high in iron. Iron attracts oxygen. Iron and oxygen work together in burning up toxic waste. There is nothing better to help remove serious disease, toxins, waste, poisons and damaged tissues from the body. It greatly helps in the elimination of mucus, acids and mucoid fecal substance from the body as well as putrifaction and bad odors. It destroys germs and harmful bacteria and is a natural and powerful antiseptic, especially for the intestinal tract. It's the best internal deodorant and blood builder there is. With any chronic or degenerative disease, I would use chlorophyll. It's a super-concentrated source of vitamins, minerals and enzymes. I prefer making it fresh, as this is its most effective form. Manual wheat grass juicers cost about $75 new. Then we can make our own "green drink," using a variety of fresh, organic herbs, diluted with distilled water. The best ingredients are alfalfa leaves, wheat grass, watercress, parsley, kale, collard, or any of the greens, comfrey leaves, plantain (herb), and dandelion. When we're not cleansing, it's also very effective with fresh beet or carrot juice. Consistently drinking one or two ounces, three or four times a day, will bring us the health and energy we've always hoped for. If everyone would use this Cleansing Program, drink fresh chlorophyll drinks, and stay away from high-protein foods, I believe that in less than 10 years there would be little disease. This is Nature's Magic, and it is going to be much more effective in a clean body that can assimilate it properly.

There are sources of liquid chlorophyll that are available at any health food store. Some are ready-made and organic. In this form, chlorophyll is an effective breath cleanser when swished around in the mouth before swallowing. Some people become ill by using liquid chlorophyll that is not organic or has flavors in it, such as mint. I suggest *DeSouza's Liquid Chlorophyll,* which is organic, or powdered chlorophyll tablets, which are excellent.

BLUE GREEN ALGAE is a very high source of vitamins, minerals, amino acids, enzymes, and chlorophyll, and is useful when the body's energy is low. It gives extra strength, endurance and support. If you feel you may be subject to a drop in energy while cleansing, it may be advisable to include it. I believe that Blue Green Algae is one of the best nutritional supplements available. Testimonies from users are impressive. Many report more energy, improvement in memory, the disappearance of various diseases; and recently, some people claim they were cured of cancer, leukemia, and AIDS. It was found that they took up to 12 to 15 grams of Blue Green Algae to obtain the desired results. I haven't had the time as yet to verify these reports.

DISTILLED WATER is definitely the best, and is strongly recommended. It only pulls from the body that which is loose, and cannot pull anything that is part of cell tissue. However, in distillation the life force is lost. You can replace it by adding some freshly-squeezed lemon, lime, or orange juice to it. Aqua Vita in Tucson, Arizona, pumps purified air into their water which completely rejuvenates it. If you can't get chlorine-free water, then at least boil it, as this will evaporate the chlorine. After it cools, it will be good for drinking and taking enemas. If it has sodium fluoride in it, then you need to get distilled water, because fluoride is a deadly poison–a by-product of the aluminum industry–and will not dissipate by boiling. Mineral water is not good because the minerals in it are *inorganic.*

FRUIT JUICE which is fresh and organically grown is best. You can make your own juice, using apples, watermelons, cantaloupe, etc. Second choice is buying juice from stores which carry fresh, organic apple juice. Third choice is purchasing organically-grown fruit juice that is pasteurized. This is readily available at any health food store. Apple is still probably the best, but berry, grape, grapefruit, orange, and occasionally, pineapple juice is fine. Juice should never contain any sugar, corn syrup, fructose or any unnatural ingredients.

Use orange juice only if you've been on the Cleanse several times, or have fasted quite a bit, and been a vegetarian for a few years. It is so cleansing that it can cause rapid elimination of toxic waste, making it difficult for the body to handle. Always dilute your juice with distilled water while on the Cleanse.

Those who feel they have Candida albicans (or anyone who does not tolerate fruit juices) should use herbal teas or just plain water to mix with the "psyllium shake". Peppermint, licorice root, hibiscus, stevia, and lemon grass are all tasty teas. Any other will do if you like it. You could use fresh vegetable juices (except carrot), but it will slow down your cleansing. Some health food stores also have a "Gourmet Psyllium Husk Powder" that helps balance the pH in the intestines. It seems to be helping those who have Candida albicans and hypoglycemia.

FLORA GROW is a non-dairy combination of micro organisms which is free from common allergens. I have investigated most of the bacteria on the market today, and have found nothing more potent or that works better for oral implants. It supplies the system with the natural bacteria for the human intestinal tract. It first creates an acid environment, restricting the growth of pathogenic organisms, and about 24 hours later, begins producing alkaline by-products. This is necessary for a healthy bowel environment. Many people are under the false assumption that acidophilus is the natural bacteria for the human body.

Lactobacillus acidophilus requires a certain nutrition to survive. I believe that it actually competes with us in terms of the food we eat. After all, when you stop to think that 25 to 35% of the fecal matter is composed of bacteria, it becomes plain that there is a great deal of substance that must be fed. It is hungry stuff. It needs folic acid, niacin, and riboflavin, to name a few of the vitamins. It uses calcium, and who doesn't have calcium problems these days? Another consideration about Lactobacillus acidophilus is the pH it produces. The optimal growth pH is between 5.5-6.2. Acidophilus begins to go dormant at a pH of 6.5. This presents a problem for our bodies. Enzymes of the small intestine cannot efficiently function at this pH; it is too acid for the body and forces it to use more organic sodium and calcium to buffer the acids created. The more acidophilus we take, the harder the body must work to compensate for the increased acids. The optimum pH range for most of the digestive enzymes in the small intestine is about 7.5. For the body to have to deal with this kind of situation causes energy drain.

Presently we use Flora Grow orally to implant the friendly bacteria in the small intestines. It is important to implant both orally and rectally immediately after the Cleanse. This product is available through some health food stores or health care practitioners.

LIQUID MINERALS are optional but *very advisable*—a wonderful product containing organic, chelated, colloidal, non-toxic minerals, which means the minerals are in a state wherein they are tiny enough to be absorbed quickly and easily through cell membranes to be utilized by the body. This product is extremely valuable for those who have not been assimilating their foods properly or who have not been on good, clean, nutritious diets. In terms of cleansing, these Liquid Minerals greatly assist the metabolic enzymes in their process of of elimination; and in terms of better health and overcoming disease, they assist the enzymes in rebuilding the body.

Reports about this product reach near-miracle levels. I've heard of gray hair returning to its natural color, and rashes, arthritis, cataracts, diabetes, and other diseases disappearing after using Liquid Minerals for an extended period of time. (However, no claims are made for the curing of these conditions by its use.) It can be applied externally on rashes, sores and bites and is excellent for burns and for the complexion. This product is considered by some doctors and nutritionists to be the most complete and effective source of organic minerals now available. It is loaded with over 60 minerals and trace minerals. People need organic minerals and most people are not getting them.

Using Liquid Minerals before, during and after the Cleanse makes for better cleansing. You don't need them to clean out the mucoid plaque, but they will help, and your body will be better for having used them. For those concerned about electrolytes, this will help, but Herbal Nutrition is better. Organic minerals usually work slowly but surely, and it is suggested that you take them for about seven weeks before you judge their effectiveness. Suggested dosage is 1 tablespoon for each 30 pounds of body weight twice a day for 2 weeks, cutting the dose in half thereafter. While cleansing, use the same amount as on your first two weeks, but divide it up into 5 equal amounts and take along with the herbs. Because of the bitter taste, you might want to take Liquid Minerals diluted with fruit or vegetable juices. Pineapple juice works well to disguise the bitter taste, and prune juice is good too. Capsules of Dehydrated Liquid Minerals are available and are much easier to take. *Warning: Liquid Minerals are less expensive, but have an acidic effect. They should be used only when a person has a full alkaline reserve.*

A SIXTEEN-OUNCE SHAKER CONTAINER will be needed for the "Psyllium Shake". Any container with a tight lid will do fine.

AN ENEMA BAG will be required. If you have a colema board or the "Ultimate Colon Unit", that would work great also.

6

DIRECTIONS FOR THE "CLEAN-ME-OUT PROGRAM"

Note: VERY IMPORTANT!
Before doing the Cleanse, first read the new
***UPDATES* that are in the back of the book.**

Pre-Cleanse Preparation — Phase III

There are three phases of the "Clean-Me-Out Program." Before doing the Cleanse it is very advisable to do a short pH test to determine if it is safe to do so. (See *UPDATES,* page 118.) Extremely acid people should not do any fasting or cleansing (except Phase III) until they have built up their alkaline reserve.

About 1 to 4 weeks before starting Phase I, **we need to do the Pre-Cleanse, as it takes time for the herbs to go into the system and condition the mucoid plaque so that it can be removed.**

When using the vegetarian Chomper and Herbal Nutrition in tablet form, plus the psyllium shakes, the mucoid plaque usually begins to be eliminated while still on the Pre-Cleanse. (Note: See "Determining the Amount of Chomper & Herbal Nutrition to be Used," under *UPDATES,* page 128.)

It is important to take at least two psyllium shakes a day while on the Pre-Cleanse and three is better. Below is the ideal Pre-Cleanse or Phase III. Eat two meals a day and take a psyllium shake three times a day. Take herbs* 1-1/2 hours after each shake and 2 hours after each meal.

6:00 am Psyllium Shake	12:00 pm Lunch	5:00 pm Herbs
7:30 am Herbs	2:00 pm Herbs	6:30 pm Dinner
9:00 am Psyllium Shake	3:30 pm Psyllium Shake	8:30 pm Herbs
10:30 am Herbs		

(Note: Never take herbs with the psyllium shake. Each will counteract the other to a large extent. *Herbs are Chomper, Herbal Nutrition, Cayenne and Dehydrated Minerals. The last two are optional. For much better results I strongly suggest also taking cayenne pepper and liquid minerals.)

It is best to take one 90,000 H.U. cayenne capsule each time the herbs are taken. (If another potency is used, take 2 capsules. One 90,000 H.U. cayenne capsule is over twice as strong as most other cayennes that are encapsulated.) The dose can be increased up to 2 or 3 if desired.

For Liquid Mineral dosage, follow the directions on the label. Increasing this dosage is also recommended. Maximum dosage *per day* is suggested. Taking as many as five is likely to cause cleansing reactions.

During the Pre-Cleanse period eat no meat, dairy products, sugar or products with sugar in them (get into the habit of reading labels), and especially no salt. Have no fried foods or foods cooked in oil. Limit your intake to olive oil and flax seed oil. Honey, real maple syrup, and date sugar sweeteners are okay. Eat all the fruit, salads and raw or cooked vegetables you want. Try to have at least one raw meal per day, and plenty of fresh vegetable juice and fresh fruit juice. If conditions in your life make this difficult, just do the best you can.

Millet is okay because it is alkaline, but limit the other grains or beans to only twice a week, and those should be soaked overnight before you lightly cook them. (Easy does it on the beans.) If you do this, you will condition your body for cleansing in a gradual way that will keep you from feeling badly, while removing excess toxins that you don't need.

The Day Before Starting the Cleanse

Your last regular meal should be lunch. The evening meal should consist of fresh, raw fruit. It is a good habit to get into— making your dinner of fresh fruit only. You will find that you sleep better at night and your body will cleanse itself while you sleep. There are some who feel that you could put a stop to one-half your ailments by doing that alone!

Take an enema two-to-three hours before going to bed. (Refer to *"How to Take an Enema"* if this is foreign territory for you. Don't knock enemas until you've read the chapter and tried one!) One hour before bed take two or more "Chomper" and three or four "Herbal Nutrition." From now on *nothing* should be eaten for seven days unless you are following *Phase II – Easy Does It.*

During the Cleanse

Drink water. Dr. Christopher suggests that in addition to fruit and vegetable juices, one should drink one ounce of distilled water daily for each pound of one's body weight. Therefore, on a regular eating diet, a person weighing 130 pounds would need 130 ounces (or one gallon) of distilled water a day. During the Cleanse, try to drink two quarts of water a day in addition to your other drinks. You can drink all the herbal teas you want as long as you use distilled water and as long as there is absolutely no black tea or sugar in it. Distilled water is important because, like bentonite, distilled water helps to extract inorganic minerals, calcium deposits and other toxic wastes from the body. Besides, as I mentioned before, it's much safer to drink than most tap water.

Some people express concern about distilled water pulling out the body's electrolytes or organic minerals. About the only time this may "appear" to happen is when someone's body is already depleted of these elements. This condition would indicate that there is a problem in digestion, assimilation, or diet. It might also indicate a malfunction of the body or an environmental problem. Dr. Walker had been drinking distilled water since 1930 and was in good health at the ripe age of 116! An interesting fact is that the liquids in fruits are identical to distilled water. That's one of the reasons why fruits are so cleansing and can succeed in repairing the body when all else fails. During the Cleanse, feel free to drink all the fresh fruit juices you like, too. (Remember the warning about fresh orange juice or other citrus juices. And remember to dilute your juice 50/50 with water!)

51

During Phase I, remember that it is a very good idea to take enemas twice every day — three or four bags in the morning and repeat two-to-three hours before bed. If conditions cause you to miss one (and you can't even make it a quick 15-minute one), increase your "Chomper" during the day to keep things moving. Five times a day, every three hours, drink the "psyllium shake". This mixture should be the first of your ten feedings during the day. (Now you can understand why you will never feel hungry.) Here's how to mix it:

- pour one or more <u>tablespoons</u> of extra thick liquid bentonite in a shake container (shake bentonite before using) NOTE: If you do not use extra thick bentonite, about six tablespoons are needed.
- add 2-4 ounces juice
- add 8-10 ounces water (distilled is best)
- add 2 <u>teaspoons</u> of psyllium husk powder
- shake briskly for five to ten seconds
- drink immediately as this mixture gels quickly (the warmer the liquid, the quicker it gels; don't make it so cold that it hurts to drink)
- drink a "chaser" of 8 ounces or more distilled water (you can flavor it with juice)

Then five times a day, one-and-a-half hours after drinking each "psyllium shake", swallow the following herbs with eight ounces of distilled water:

- 2 or more "Chomper"
- 3 or 4 "Herbal Nutrition"
- Optional but highly recommended: Power-Up (1 or more)

Fifteen minutes before taking the herbs, take the Liquid Minerals (optional) in a small amount of fruit juice. Your last "feeding" of the day should be the herbs. On this last feeding, add one or more extra "Chomper".

Stay on Schedule

Schedule yourself to take the feedings at regular, hour-and-a-half intervals and stick to your schedule (to avoid feeling weak at any time). You can start as early as you like. Just make sure you get all ten feedings in. Here's an example of a schedule you might follow:

> 7:00 am—Psyllium Shake
> 8:30 am—Herbs & Chlorophyll* (take enema #1)
> 10:00 am—Psyllium Shake
> 11:30 am—Herbs & Chlorophyll*
> 1:00 pm—Psyllium Shake
> 2:30 pm—Herbs & Chlorophyll*
> 4:00 pm—Psyllium Shake
> 5:30 pm—Herbs & Chlorophyll* (take enema #2)
> 7:00 pm—Psyllium Shake
> 8:30 pm—Herbs (add a "Chomper") & Chlorophyll*

> * Power-Up can be substituted for Chlorophyll each time.

Directions for Phase II—Easy Does It
(The Easy Way to Cleanse)

Absolutely anyone can do Phase II. This is designed for those who are addicted to eating. If you're one whose salivary glands seem overactive and whose stomach growls every time you see food or even pictures of food—this program is for you.

Phase II - Easy Does It is also designed for those who are extremely toxic, those who are very weak physically and those whose aches and pains are such that it would keep them from cleansing. The elderly and those with serious diseases should be on this program.

During *Phase II - Easy Does It* follow the same directions given for *Phase I - Go For It* for one or two days, depending on your condition. Around noon on the third through seventh days, eat one meal of the following: raw salad, fresh fruits, lightly steamed vegetables or some baked potatoes. Stay away from everything else that is cooked or processed.

In every other respect, this program is exactly like *Phase I - Go For It*. You will simply consider this meal one of your feedings (a substitute for the "psyllium shake"). One-and-a-half hours later you will be back on schedule, taking your herbs and chlorophyll. Make sure you still get in your other nine feedings.

Phase II – Easy Does It can be done by anyone and will still eliminate mucoid matter and toxins. It just keeps the body from doing it faster than you might be comfortable with. Therefore, do not expect to eliminate the same 25-50 feet of mucoid matter that those on *Phase I – Go For It* can expect to pass. But do expect to rid your body of the toxic substances—just at a slower rate. Some are still removing 15-25 feet a week doing the Cleanse this way, which is still more than one can eliminate following the other cleanses on the market.

Cleansing Reactions

One well-known colon cleansing program claims no cleansing reactions. I tried it. Not only did I feel terrible for a month, but I got absolutely nothing out. Now depending on the toxicity of the body, there may be cleansing reactions, which will differ from person to person. Most people never feel bad while on the Cleanse, but some do. However, I no longer recommend that people just "tough it out," even though you may really want results (See page 66 for an update on cleansing reactions).

The older or weaker the person is, or the more foul the intestinal tract, the more likely there will be cleansing reactions. Realize that the more cleansing reactions you have, the more your body is crying out to be cleansed. Cleansing reactions may reveal themselves as skin eruptions or in the very symptoms of the disease you are trying to get rid of. My wife had gone on the Cleanse about five times in a seven-month period. On her third cleanse (having never had any cleansing reactions before), she finished the seven days as usual and then, for the first time, began to eat raw fruits and vegetables only. (She usually would just go back to her regular diet, which included some cooked foods). Then the cleansing reactions set in. She had every symptom of the walking pneumonia and bronchitis she had suffered in her childhood and early 20's. However, this time she rejoiced, for she knew that she was ridding herself of those symptoms forever. After ten days of telling herself and certain well-meaning individuals (who kept insisting that she had abused her body with "that fast") that she was just experiencing a valuable "healing crisis," her health returned. Before that cleanse, every time she exercised or even climbed stairs she would wheeze and feel a heavy congestion being stirred up in her chest. After that ten-day period, those symptoms disappeared and now they do not recur even when she's backpacking or playing tennis.

You may experience other reactions such as dizziness or spaciness. People with the increasingly-popular candida albicans (which I am beginning to suspect could be related to parasites, but which is being diagnosed as a yeast infection) often feel weak or tired while cleansing. If you fall into this category, again, see page 66. I had candida, and during the first ten cleanses I felt terrible— well, not all that bad, but weak. Each time after finishing any cleanse, the candida symptoms lessened. After my second time on the "Clean-Me-Out Program" I experienced almost no cleansing reactions and felt better on the Cleanse than while eating. This is probably attributable to the fact that I was getting cleaner and cleaner with each cleansing.

Meat eaters have more reactions than vegetarians only because, as a rule, they have more filth to get rid of (see page 102). Most everyone else will have no problems at all (unless they have had a lot of drugs or sugar). Occasionally a very toxic mucoid layer may loosen from the intestinal wall and its debris will flood the system with temporary toxic waste. If this happens you may feel nauseous and weak. That's the time for an extra enema or colonic—this helps to move it out fast. As soon as that toxic substance comes out, you'll feel better immediately.

Something like this happened to me once on the fourth day of my first cleanse when I was sitting in front of the fireplace reading a book. I had been feeling fine. Then suddenly, I felt something shift in my abdomen and I started to feel weak, then worse and worse. I put the book down and slumped in the chair. I could hardly move. About 40 minutes went by when I felt the urge to go to the bathroom. I made it to the bathroom and sat down—it flew out! I looked in the toilet and couldn't believe my eyes. It was the longest and most spectacular piece of hardened mucoid gunk I had ever seen — *two feet long* and very dark. It gave me great encouragement to keep on cleansing. But what was more, I felt fantastic. I went into the other room and for the first time in years I felt like doing push-ups. (And did them!)

With the very sick, elderly or weak, caution is advised. Almost everyone needs to eliminate more, but some are too weak to do so. When we begin to use cleansing herbs, the body may click into gear and start eliminating from anywhere and everywhere, causing what to some would be alarming symptoms. These individuals should ease into herbal programs more cautiously (following *Phase II – Easy Does It*) and under the supervision of a health professional who has a lot of experience in herbal cleansing as well as the equipment to test the body's conditions. If you can find such a rare health professional you will be fortunate indeed. Their successes being so high, they are under constant suspicion and the watchful eye of the A.M.A. In fact, the moment they have even a tiny slip-up, they are locked up immediately. Many of the great healers or promoters of alternative approaches to health have been put in jail—Christoper, Irons and others. Dr. Shook disappeared suddenly and was presumed murdered.

The Tongue

You will notice as you cleanse that your tongue will turn white and filmy and your breath will be foul. This is somewhat a reflection of what is happening inside the digestive canal. As you use the herbs and drink the juice, the mucoid layers will soften some. You may notice that your abdomen swells. As more and more mucoid layers are removed, the swelling will go down. Your tongue will become more and more clear. This is a good gauge as to how clean you are becoming. For when you are all cleaned out, your tongue will be shining red (just like a newborn baby's). It will be free of all whiteness or film and your breath will be permanently sweet. Even your bowel movements will become sweet-smelling (this may also occur during the Cleanse). If you eat poorly—odors will return. Let this be your goal: to be sweet-smelling from one end to the other!

How to Stop the Cleanse

(*Note:* Take 4-6 "Chomper" the evening of the 6th day to push things through, and schedule your Cleanse so that you'll be free the morning of the 8th day for an implant of Flora Grow.)

On the morning of the 7th day of the Cleanse, prepare the oral implant to be taken that evening: Break open and empty 2 capsules of Flora Grow into 6 oz. of spring or mineral water (unchlorinated, uncarbonated and *not distilled*) and let stand for 8-12 hours. Do not take any psyllium shakes after 3:00 p.m. In their place drink any type of fresh juice, unless Candidiasis is present. Fresh carrot juice is delicious. If you are really hungry after this, eat some fruit. Continue taking the herbs, increasing the number of "Chomper" by 2-4. You are preparing for the implantation of Flora Grow, and your objective at this point is to clean the intestines of the bulk substance so that it will not interfere with the implant. In the evening, drink fresh juice for supper. One hour later take more herbs, increasing "Chomper" as above, and sometime in the evening take a regular enema then drink the Flora Grow preparation that was made in the morning.

To prepare for the following morning's rectal implant, empty the contents of 4 capsules of Flora Grow into 16 oz. of spring or mineral water, and let stand for 8-12 hours or overnight. Also, prepare another 2 capsules for the next morning's oral implant.

On the morning of the 8th day drink the Flora Grow mixture then take a thorough enema. Don't rush it. You could also take a colonic or use the "Ultimate Colon Unit," as long as no chemicals (such as chlorine) are in the water. If you've been using tap water for enemas, switch to distilled water—at least for the last gallon—as chlorine destroys the good bacteria. If you took enough "Chomper," all the bulk should have passed through by the end of the enema.

While waiting 2 hours, have breakfast. Any fresh fruit in season would be good. Do not mix fruits, especially melons and citrus. Two hours or more after the end of the enema you may feel that more loosened mucoid substance or bulk needs to be expelled. If so, take another enema and wait 2 more hours. If not, proceed with the implant.

Implantation Procedure

• Pour the Flora Grow mixture made the night before into the enema bag. If the enemas are taken on the back, place a pillow under the hips to elevate them and help the liquid to remain inside.

• Let the mixture enter slowly and use the hands to move it up the descending colon, across the transverse and down the ascending colon by massaging the abdomen.

• Once the entire 16 oz. is in, roll over onto the right side, again massaging the liquid to the furthest end of the colon.

• Retain the liquid as long as possible. Should you feel the need to eliminate, lift the hips higher and stay in this position until the urge passes. As long as the mixture is retained even for a few minutes, you will receive many of its benefits.

• If you should experience any gas, take another small enema, using distilled water. This will allow the gas to escape and relax the colon. Keep in mind that the colon has just had its pH chemistry changed, which is why the body sometimes produces gas and other slight reactions, which will soon pass.

• In the evening and the following morning repeat the above implantation procedure, remembering that the longer the Flora Grow mixture is retained, the more effective the implant.

More About Ending the Cleanse

Lunch should consist of either fresh fruit or lightly-steamed vegetables, freshly-made soup, or a raw salad with natural lemon juice dressing, if you wish. Whenever you eat out, bring your own olive oil (*please, never use safflower or corn oil*), and apple cider vinegar or lemon. Restaurant salad dressings are often 50% sugar. The oils they use are extremely hard on the liver, and their vinegar is distilled, which is also destructive to the body, and contains dye.

Supper should consist of fresh, raw fruit. Eat all you want. Two hours after supper take some more "Chomper." Immediately before bed take the oral implant and prepare another oral implant for next morning. Take the last rectal implant and if possible, retain it all night.

The 9th day's menu should be fruit for breakfast, salad, vegetable soup, or lightly steamed vegetables for lunch, and a supper of whatever you feel is best. I would suggest fresh fruit.

From here on out, your diet is up to you. Try not to overeat or be influenced by old desires for unhealthy cooked foods.

Oral Implants: It is best to take 1 capsule of Flora Grow twice a day, morning and evening (2 per day), for 2 weeks. Then take one capsule a day until bottle runs out. (Soak it in mineral water or spring water for maximum results. If this is not convenient, it will work by just swallowing the capsule.)

Note: Best to take it first thing in the morning or 30 minutes to one hour before bed on an empty stomach. Taking it about 30 minutes before a meal is okay. If time is a problem, you can take right after a meal when the hydrochloric acid is in its most diluted state.

Those who suspect that they have Candidiasis, E-Coli, or a predominance of other unfriendly bacteria, should begin taking Yeast End 2 weeks after starting the Flora Grow. It is necessary to build up the bacteria before using Yeast End (see page 130).

Should Constipation Occur: It is customary to become constipated for about 2 days just after the Cleanse. About 40 to 60% of the normal stool is composed of bacteria and it takes several days to build that up again. After the bacteria has grown back, bowel movements should be normal. Those who are usually constipated may find their problem is ended even after the first Cleanse, and the bacteria re-established. If not, they should take one psyllium shake a day, without bentonite. This will supply the needed fiber to keep things moving.

After the end of the second day, anyone who has not had a bowel movement, should take some Chomper and Herbal Nutrition that evening. The next morning they should start taking one psyllium shake (without bentonite) a day for several days and use Chomper and Herbal Nutrition only as needed. It is best not to rely upon these herbs unless there is a problem.

Suggestions

Some people use Chomper and Herbal Nutrition on a regular basis until their digestive systems are working normally. The herbs in Chomper are not true laxatives. They clean, feed, stimulate, and rebuild the lining and peristaltic muscles of the stomach and small intestines. Keep in mind that while the formula or combination is relatively new, the herbs are natural, time-tested, and are able to work with the body's natural, self-healing abilities. This is not at all like taking drugstore laxatives, which are both harmful and habit-forming.

It is important to understand that these herbs are designed to remove the mucoid plaque. They are not designed to work as a laxative. People who need a laxative and are not using these herbs to eliminate the mucoid plaque, should try having extra fiber and plenty of water in their diets. People are surprised to find how well their digestive system will work by drinking one very large glass of water first thing in the morning. If that doesn't do it, then they should try one psyllium shake without bentonite in the morning, after they drink their water.

Do not take any more psyllium and bentonite shakes until two or three days after you have finished the entire bottle of Flora Grow. The reason for this is that you want to allow time for friendly bacteria to be well-established. Just taking psyllium without bentonite will not cause a problem.

Once you're certain that you have a good implant (and you will know this because bowel movements will be easy, soft, and have no unpleasant odor), more mucoid layers can be removed by doing Phase III (see *UPDATES*, page 128 and 129) as long as you like.

Try to eat only two meals a day (not including fruits). Eat fruit for snacks either one-half hour before meals or three or more hours after meals. Pineapple or apples are the only fruits I would eat after regular meals. (They are digestive aids!)

As long as you are regulating your dosage of Chomper, 1-2 feet of mucoid fecal layers may continue to pass out every day.

Note: Unless you are on Phase I or II of the "Clean-Me-Out Program" it is best to take occasional breaks from the herbs so that the body does not become immune to their healing effects. I would suggest that with any herbs, you take them for six days and go off the seventh. Then take them (if you feel your body needs them) for six weeks and go off of them the seventh week, etc. In this manner they will continue to give your body their maximum benefits.

7

HOW TO TAKE AN ENEMA

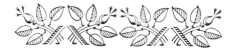

"Think not that it is sufficient that the angel of water embrace you outwards only. I tell you truly, the uncleanness within is greater by much than the uncleanness without. And he who cleanses himself without, but within remains unclean, is like to tombs that outwards are painted fair, but are within full of all manner of horrible uncleanness and abominations."

"Seek, therefore, a large trailing gourd, having a stalk the length of a man; take out its inwards and fill it with water from the river which the sun has warmed. Hang it upon a branch of a tree, and kneel upon the ground before the angel of water, and suffer the end of the stalk of the trailing gourd to enter your hinder parts, that the water may flow through all your bowels. Afterwards rest kneeling on the ground before the angel of water that he will free your body from every uncleanness and disease. Then let the water run out from your body, that it may carry away from within all the unclean and evil-smelling things of Satan. And you shall see with your eyes and smell with your nose all the abominations and uncleanness which defiled the temple of your body; even all the sins which abode in your body, tormenting you with all manner of pains."

(*Gospel of Peace of Jesus Christ* by the Disciple John)

Learn to appreciate and enjoy enemas. Nothing short of Divine Intervention (also known as miracles) can come to your rescue faster to relieve you of pressure, headaches, constipation, various pains, gas and massive accumulations of toxic mucus, pus and poisonous waste.

Some people are downright afraid to take enemas. This is generally due to either embarrassment or lack of knowledge. Anything this good for you should not be embarrassing. Taking enemas is wise and intelligent until one is completely pure inside. They are fully constructive, lifting you to a higher level of existence through purification. If you are going to be embarrassed, consider being embarrassed by the things you do which are destructive to your Temple—like drinking alcoholic beverages, coffee and pop, eating meat, sugar and dairy products, eating more than you need, swearing or being overweight.

On the other hand, you simply may not know how to take one. Don't let that stop you. It's easy to learn. Be brave! Consider it a new dimension of living yet to be explored. A vast, new frontier of experience awaits you! I guarantee you it will become the most enjoyable part of the Cleanse—seeing the results of your efforts coming out of you in living color!

When on the Cleanse, taking enemas twice daily will usually help a person rid himself of an extra ten feet of mucoid layers in a seven-day period. I know a friend who refused to take enemas during the Cleanse. Being an herbalist, he figured that if he took extra cascara sagrada he could keep things moving and avoid enemas completely. But there were times when he did not feel good—a clear indication that toxic substance was being stirred up and needed to be released. He would have had relief had he taken enemas. The next time he went on the Cleanse, he decided to go with the enemas. He overcame his aversion to them very quickly when he saw the benefits. His cleansing went much easier and he now recommends enemas to everyone doing the Cleanse.

Without exception, everyone I have seen go on this Cleanse without taking enemas has had a worse-than-average time of it. So, I would say that if you won't take enemas during the Cleanse— forget it. Don't bother cleansing. When you become really miserable and your friend, Mr. Pain, brings you to your senses, your silly embarrassment or lack of knowledge will be something you will want to conquer, instead of letting it conquer you.

Equipment Needed

I recommend a douche bag instead of the tiny enema bags you find in the drug stores. They are easier and faster to use. They are also less expensive. If you get the douche bag, spend a dollar and get the enema tip to replace the douche tip, although either will work.

Olive oil (or any lubricant) is placed on the tip of the enema and on the anus for easy injection. Any kind of salad oil is okay, but olive oil is very healing and purifying - in addition to being good for most rashes. (We generally use that or most any liquid oil from a health food store.) You will need a gallon jug to fill the douche bag. You can use any size container, but the gallon jug makes it easier and faster to use.

What to Use for Enema Liquid

Most of the time, I use just plain old tap water. But in some areas of the country I would not. In Mt. Shasta, the water is just about as pure as it can get. In Chicago, I wouldn't even consider it. Distilled water is good. Purified water is fine. Sometimes, about halfway through the Cleanse, I use herbal teas. One teaspoon of herbs per gallon of water works well. Make the tea and then filter. The following herbs make excellent enemas:

CATNIP has a soothing effect on the body; good for energy; improves circulation; excellent for colds, fever, gas and especially good for children or those who have trouble taking enemas.

BURDOCK ROOT is one of the best blood purifiers you'll find; the best herb for skin; improves kidney action and helps eliminate calcium deposits.

YARROW is one of the better herbs; good for the liver, stomach and glands; a blood purifier, it opens the pores of the skin (the body's largest elimination organ) for rapid elimination; good for colds, cramps, fever and flu; also good to take a bath in.

RED RASPBERRY is excellent for all kinds of female problems; high in iron, it is good for the eyes and for elimination; it is very nutritious.

Other excellent enema herbs are blessed thistle, plantain, pleurisy root, thyme, hyssop, mint, elder flower, white oak bark, yellow dock, mullein, echinacea, dandelion, parsley, marshmallow root and peppermint. Though I sometimes use more than one herb (such as 2-3 capsules of my "Herbal Bright Eyes" formula which works wonders on my eyes), I would say that unless you consider yourself an herbalist, *beware of combinations.*

Temperature of Enema Liquid

The hotter the liquid, the faster it will be absorbed through the colon. The muscles will relax and this is not what you want. I prefer the temperature to be right at body temperature or a little cooler. The muscles will stay strong at this tepid temperature for maximum evacuation.

To awaken and bring strength to the peristaltic muscles in the colon use cooler or cold water for your last gallon of enema liquid (it is best to do this after you feel you have gotten all of the loose matter out of the colon with a gallon or so of lukewarm water first). You will feel a wonderful sensation down in the colon that will strengthen the whole lower abdomen.

Injection Procedure

NOTE: When putting liquid in enema bag, be sure the valve is shut. After you've sprayed your feet and clean bathroom with an herbal tea enema the first time, you won't have to remind yourself of this!

Place the filled enema bag on the shower or bathroom door handle, or on the towel rack. This is a comfortable height. After you get used to enemas, feel free to hang it higher—remember that the higher you hang the bag, the more pressure there is and the liquid will flow out faster. You can control the flow with the enema bag shut-off valve, which is about two inches from the tip.

Put the lubricant on the enema tip and on the anus. Place the tip over the toilet, sink or bathtub and open the valve, allowing the liquid to flow until the air bubbles are removed from the tube. Then get into position (after shutting off the valve) and insert. After insertion, open the valve gradually, allowing the liquid to flow up the colon slowly until you get used to it. Always keep your hand on the valve for quick shut-off when needed and to keep the tip from slipping out (unless you are using the douche tip).

Position for the Enema

Some people prefer laying on the back—this way they are in a good position to be comfortable and massage the colon. I like to be on my knees with my head on a towel. To me, it feels like the liquid flows to the furthest end of the colon much easier than when I'm on my back. When I want to be very thorough, I not only massage the colon (while the liquid is in) in that position, but also on my back and on both sides before getting up to eliminate. While some may not choose to massage at all, you can figure that the more you massage the colon, the more will come out.

Starting with the descending colon (left side of the lower abdomen), work up to the transverse (just behind the lower rib cage, unless you have a prolapsus) and then down the ascending colon (right side). Work it well—get the liquid all the way down to the ileocecal. If you aren't sure where all these parts of the colon are, just massage the heck out of your lower abdomen. Then go to the toilet and release! Be prepared to be amazed and astounded at what will come out of you. Now you will begin to enjoy enemas. Keep in mind that, depending on your pre-cleanse preparation, you may not get any of the ''real stuff'' out until your third day.

In times when the liquid has difficulty flowing up into the colon it helps considerably to take deep breaths—all the way in and all the way out. This changes the pressure in the abdomen area and makes it easier for the liquid to pass through.

How Much Liquid

When you first begin the enema you may get a cup or so in, depending upon how compacted you are. That's okay—don't force it. As soon as the pressure gets uncomfortable, shut off the valve. Try to work the liquid past the congestion by massaging as indicated above; then add more liquid. You will know when it's too much. Then evacuate. You should pass some blockages. Let it all out, then do it again. This time you will get more in. Although you may never reach it, make a goal of continuing the procedure until you can get the whole bag (2 quarts) in. Keep doing this until chunks stop coming out. Who would want putrifying toxic garbage in their bodies even a second longer than it has to be? I recommend going through two gallons. If you've got a time shortage, remember that a shorter enema is infinitely better than no enema. And you'll be a *lot* more comfortable wherever you're going if you take that extra time for your enema before you go.

I would recommend you take your two enemas first thing in the morning and at five or six in the evening. If you do it before bed you may have to get up during the night, since the liquid is often left in the colon and gradually seeps into the kidneys. If you are urinating too often, chew some juniper berries. You may want to take juniper berry powder instead. This will break up uric acid deposits and clean the urinary system. It will also help relax the bladder. After taking juniper for a day or two, you will experience how much it assists in sleeping through the night. Using juniper tea can make that happen even sooner.

An Update on Cleansing Reactions

Nobody needs to feel bad while cleansing. If people experience discomfort for more than a few hours, then they should SLOW DOWN THE CLEANSE BY GOING BACK TO PHASE II OR PHASE III! I've discovered that it's not a good idea to "tough it out" when we are going through really rough cleansing reactions. Most people are extremely toxic. If we haven't prepared ourselves enough by doing longer "Pre-Cleanses" (Phase III), we should be more careful and not try to hurry into greater health. After all, we spent our entire life polluting ourselves, so why should we be in such an all-fired rush and put ourselves through unnecessary suffering just to get cleaned out in record time? That kind of punishment may result in not wanting to do any more cleansing, and that decision may result in years of poor health, low energy, chronic disease, unnecessary unhappiness and an early death.

Many of us have seen such incredible results using the "Clean-Me-Out Program", that others are excited about achieving similar results - so they become willing to grit their teeth when the going gets rough. Although I greatly admire these kinds of people, I no longer believe in forcing ourselves through the tough times, because the toxins, mucus, fungus, chemicals and other poisons are finally getting out, but faster than our bodies can handle. That may put too much stress on the kidneys, liver and heart.

We can obtain our goals and never feel sluggish, tired or stressed– in fact, we really should not cleanse in any other way. Here are a few hints on what to do to prevent having to "tough it out":
1. Most people should do a long Pre-Cleanse.
2. When going on the Phase I Program and cleansing reactions become too much and they last more than a few hours, take a coffee enema. I have discovered that this can really work to our benefit, if we do it correctly. Headaches, lack of energy or just feeling terrible, could indicate that the liver is unable to handle the overload of excessive toxins. A coffee enema can cause the liver to produce more bile, opening the bile ducts and causing the bile to flow. In this process, a toxic liver can dump many of its toxins into the bile and get rid of them in just a few minutes. This can give great relief and also help against spasms, precordial (heart, throat, chest) pain and difficulties resulting from the sudden withdrawal of all sedations, alcohol and tobacco.

    Ask the people where you purchased this book where to write for directions to the coffee enema and be sure to use only organically grown coffee. (Also refer to the address on page 110.)
3. If that doesn't work, then go back to Phase III, and after feeling better, go on to Phase II or stay on Phase III for awhile.

8

EATING FOR GOOD HEALTH

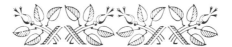

In a few years, the scientific world will be forced to announce that the natural food for man is raw fruits, raw vegetables, sprouted seeds, grains, legumes, nuts, and herbs. The Bible tells us this (Genesis 1:29), yet how many students of the Bible have the determination to overcome lustful habits of eating? This leads to rationalizing. It is not my intent to criticize those who rationalize their poor eating habits, but to encourage them to break out of those habits which are making them sick and prematurely old. Investigation of the anatomy of the human body with particular attention to the digestive processes proves, beyond any doubt, what we should and should not eat. When we eat unnatural foods, we are poisoning ourselves. The system gets overworked and, eventually, breaks down. Sugar, pop, coffee, alcohol, fried foods and preservatives and chemicals in food are poisons. Pasteurized dairy products, meat, cooked foods and wheat are poisonous to most people and over-work the body.

Avoid Dairy Products

Pasteurized cow's milk in any form is the most mucus-forming of all foods. Cow's milk is NOT the same as human milk. It is totally unnatural to man. Its imbalanced minerals react unfavorably in the body. Because it contains too much phosphorous, it is actually a poor source of calcium. When pasteurized, it has nothing in it that is of use to the body, since pasteurizing depletes milk of its enzymes, vitamins and life force. *Even a calf will die after six months on pasteurized milk.* Do you think you and your children can live any better on pasteurized cow's milk than the calf for which the milk was originally designed?

Those who must use dairy products should use those made with *raw* goat's milk since it is nearer to human milk and much less mucus-forming.

Avoid Meat

The digestive system of the meat-eating animal is completely different than man's. Its whole digestive tract is only twelve feet long. When meat has to travel through 30 feet of the human's digestive tract before it comes out the other end (if at all), it is no wonder that the meat-eater's fecal matter and gas are so foul-smelling, especially when compared to the cleaned-out vegetarian's. The meat-eater's digestion requires ten times more hydrochloric acid than can be provided by the body and most people tend to be deficient in hydrochloric acid as it is.

Early Greeks, Egyptians, Hebrews and Buddhists were all vegetarians. The Bible states: *"and God said, 'Behold, I have given you every herb-bearing seed which is upon the face of the Earth, and every tree, in which are fruits; for you it shall be as meat.'"* (Genesis 1:29) And in Ezekiel 47:12 we read *"and the fruit thereof shall be for meat, and the leaf (herbs) thereof for medicine."* St. Paul also said, *"It is good not to eat flesh."* (Romans 14:21)

In *The Gospel of Peace of Jesus Christ* by the disciple John (which was taken from the secret archives of the Vatican and from which I quote frequently in this book), Jesus says *"And the flesh of slain beasts in a person's body will become his own tomb. For I tell you truly, he who kills, kills himself and whoever eats the flesh of slain beasts eats the body of death."*

Does it seem a mystery that those who read and study the Bible continue to order the death of innocent animals by buying it from their local supermarkets and restaurants? The Bible is clear on the issue. And only when Moses spoke to his disobedient people—only for that determined disobedience was the exception made. The seeming mystery is no mystery at all. Religious faiths are too easily molded to the desires, weaknesses and appetites of their followers.

"Kill not, neither eat the flesh of your innocent prey, lest you become the slaves of Satan . . . Then another said: 'Moses, the greatest in Israel, suffered our forefathers to eat the flesh of unclean beasts. Why, therefore, do you forbid us the flesh of all beasts? Which law comes from God? That of Moses, or your law?'

"And Jesus answered: 'God gave, by Moses, ten commandments to your forefathers. "These commandments are hard," said your forefathers, and they could not keep them. When Moses saw this, he had compassion on his people, and would not that they perish. And then he gave them ten times ten commandments, less hard, that they might follow them. I tell you truly, if your forefathers had been able to keep the ten commandments of God, Moses would never had need of his ten times ten commandments. *For he whose feet are strong as the mountain of Zion, needs no crutches; but he whose limbs do shake, gets further having crutches, than without them.* And Moses said to the Lord: "My heart is filled with sorrow, for my people will be lost. For they are without knowledge, and are not able to understand thy commandments. They are as little children who cannot yet understand their father's words. Suffer, Lord, that I give them other laws, that they may not perish. If they may not be with thee, Lord, let them not be against thee; that they may sustain themselves, and when the time has come, and they are ripe for thy words, reveal to them thy laws." For that did Moses break the two tablets of stone ten times ten in their stead. And of these ten times ten the Scribes and Pharisees have made a hundred times ten commandments. And they have laid unbearable burdens on your shoulders, that they themselves do not carry. For the more nigh are the commandments to God, the less do we need; and the farther they are from God, then the more do we need. Wherefore are the laws of the Pharisees and Scribes innumerable; the laws of the Son of Man seven; of the angels three; and of God one.

'Therefore, I teach you only those laws which you can understand, that you may become men, and follow the seven laws of the Son of Man. Then will the angels also reveal their laws to you, that God's holy spirit may descend upon you, and lead you to his law.'

And all were astonished at his wisdom, and asked him: 'Continue, Master, and teach us all the laws which we can receive.'

And Jesus continued: 'God commanded your forefathers: "Thou shalt not kill." But their heart was hardened and they killed. Then Moses desired *that at least* they should not kill men, and he suffered them to kill beasts. And then the heart of your forefathers was hardened yet more, and they killed men and beasts likewise. But I do say to you: Kill neither men, nor beasts, nor yet the food which goes into your mouth. For if you eat living food, the same will quicken, but if you kill your food, the dead food will kill you also. *For life comes only from life,* and from death comes always death. For everything which kills your food, kills your bodies also. And everything which kills your bodies kills your souls also. And your bodies become what your foods are, even as your spirits, likewise, become what your thoughts are. *Therefore, eat not anything which fire, or frost, or water has destroyed. For burned, frozen and rotted foods will burn, freeze and rot your body also.* Be not like the foolish husbandman who sowed in his ground cooked, and frozen, and rotten seeds. And great was his distress. But be like that husbandman who sowed in his field living seed, and whose field bore living ears of wheat, paying a hundredfold for the seeds which he planted. For I tell you truly, live only by the fire of life, and prepare not your foods with the fire of death, which kills your foods, your bodies and your souls also.' ''

(*The Gospel of Peace of Jesus Christ* by the Disciple John)

Science used to support the consumption of meat. It no longer does. It cannot. The facts are so overwhelming that the eating of animal flesh is doomed as the age of enlightened people is ushered in. One day mankind will look back in horror at the carnivorous habits of its predecessors. Habits of meat-eating will seem as barbarian and disgusting to future man as the eating of cat and dog meat now seems to the average American. Consider these facts:

- In 1961, the Journal of the American Medical Association reported that a vegetarian diet can prevent 90-97% of heart diseases.

- Studies reveal 50% less cancer among people who eat small amounts of meat, compared to average meat eaters.

- Scotland has the highest rate of bowel cancer in the world and they eat 20% more meat than the English.

- The kidney of the meat eater must work three times harder than the kidney of the vegetarian.

- Although meat needs to get through the digestive tract fast, it takes four times longer than grains or vegetables to get through.

- During World War I, Norway and Denmark could not get meat. The death rate dropped 17% and then returned to normal when they returned to their meat diets.

- In a study of 50,000 vegetarians, the American National Institute of Health found that vegetarians live longer, have far less heart disease and a much lower cancer rate compared to meat eaters. (Note: Most American vegetarians were once meat eaters and even after many years carry old, dead meat or its toxins in their intestinal tracts as it takes serious cleansing to get rid of it. Lifelong vegetarians have a tremendous advantage, even if they eat poorly, as many do.)

- In England, vegetarians pay less for life insurance.

- Studies show that vegetarians are stronger, more agile, have greater endurance and recover from fatigue faster than meat eaters.

- A Yale University study revealed that vegetarians have nearly twice the stamina of meat eaters.

- World starvation is well-connected to meat-eating habits. If Americans stopped feeding grain to cattle, the excess grain could feed 500 million people (not to mention the land that could be used to grow food instead of being used for grazing cattle).

I was flying from L.A. to Seattle one time and was seated next to a young German lady. When a stewardess asked Rich Anderson to identify himself, I pushed the button. The lady asked me what it was about and I explained that it was for my vegetarian meal. She said she ate meat and asked why I didn't. I said, "I like animals." (Lots easier than going into mucoid-fecal-matter conversation and, besides, it's true.) She said, "So do I!" I looked at her in disbelief and said, "You do?" She got the message and just sat there, looking stunned, for several minutes. I suppose other people love animals in different ways—some love them to eat; others just love them.

Is It Easy to Suddenly Become a "Rawfooder"?

For some, maybe. I admit it wasn't easy for me. In fact, I still eat things I shouldn't. I enjoy it going down, have immediate regrets and take "Chomper" to get rid of it as soon as possible. But I keep on improving my diet.

The problem with going on a raw food diet without cleansing is this: when the average person goes on raw foods, even for just a few days, he begins to cleanse the cell structure (not the intestinal tract). That isn't going to clean out the mucoid layers, but raw foods will do serious cleansing. Eventually, it might even loosen the mucoid layers. What's wrong with that? Well, one must be very careful. The average person is so full of toxic waste that a complete raw food diet (without complete intestinal cleansing) could stir up more problems than he could handle. Fruits are the most cleansing of all. Vegetables do not cleanse nearly as rapidly. It is ironic that because of severe cleansing reactions it would sometimes appear that eating fresh, raw food makes a person sick, while eating cooked or junk foods makes a person well. All that has happened, however, is that the eating of junk foods has stopped the cleansing process.

Cleansing reactions on a raw food diet, without cleansing the digestive tract first can be so severe for the average person that a lack of energy, spaciness, eruptions of the skin, overloaded kidneys, liver and other organs can weaken him to the point of ineffectiveness. I read of one case of death actually occurring because a person was exceptionally toxic and ate raw fruit only for a long period of time. This is, unfortunately, why many who have studied health became discouraged when experimenting with the raw food diet and even concluded that raw foods were bad!

Thus, I recommend that we *first* cleanse the intestines, then work on the internal cell structure. Once the digestive system is repaired, you will be strong enough to cleanse the rest of the body. Cleansing should be done gradually and carefully. This is why I occasionally suggest eating a baked potato to those having *extreme* cleansing reactions on Phase I of the "Clean-Me-Out Program." It instantaneously stops the internal cleansing and they feel better immediately. Whenever possible, however, I would still prefer that a person suffering those reactions first try an enema. I spent 20 years trying to cleanse the cell structure of my body first. I fasted a great deal, although I did not always eat the way I should have between the fasts. I did quite well until an accident kept me from exercising (which gets rid of toxins but should become unnecessary once one is thoroughly cleaned out). Then it was downhill, with occasional ups during my fasts. Eventually I learned to cleanse the intestinal tract and my health has skyrocketed up!

What to Expect as Your Intestinal Tract Becomes Purer

Pure, clear, clean, calm water perfectly reflects the sun. Put a drop of black dye in it and observe the contrast. Then try red, brown, yellow, etc. Keep doing this for some time and two things will happen: there will be no more reflection of the sun and any further drops will cause little or no contrast. There are two points here: 1) purity is required to reflect the light, and 2) when the body is filled with filth from eating "non-foods" (anything but raw-fruits, raw vegetables, and sprouted seeds, nuts and grains) there is little noticeable affect when we eat dead foods. But when our bodies become more pure, we begin to notice the effects of the dead foods much more strongly.

My wife and I decided to experiment with that contrast. After a great deal of intestinal cleansing and a couple of months on raw foods (mostly fruit), we went back to eating the average American diet, minus meat for four days. Each morning it became more and more difficult to get out of bed, let alone feel good. We each began to develop the world's worst case of baggy eyes until by the fourth morning we had pouches instead of bags. Wrinkles in the face became decidedly more pronounced. My vision became more and more fuzzy but taking my "Herbal Bright Eyes" eye formula brought them back. Tiny little bumps developed on our skin (as the body made its desperate attempt to eliminate the toxic overload). Our complexions became dull and lifeless. We noticed that our love for each other lessened. Our sleep was interrupted by weird dreams. Our whole bodies became puffy—but it was especially noticeable in the face. The energy level became lower and lower and for the first time in years we found ourselves getting sleepy during the day. I felt some pain in my kidneys and we both experienced inflammation in various joints. We felt congested in our sinuses and throats as well as various aches and pains throughout the body. My memory became less effective. We both found it difficult to turn our attention to God. Our appetites for food became almost uncontrollable and we were hungry when we shouldn't be. Work became work, instead of the joy it usually is for us. We experienced feelings of low self-esteem and a lack of confidence. We had puffy stomachs. Our mental efficiency lessened and we became more and more prone to negative feelings. We were easily irritated and rather short-tempered. Our bodies developed foul odors that had gone away a long time ago. Being neither TV-watchers nor movie-goers, we were amazed when we actually felt the desire for such entertainment.

Believe me, we were so happy to get back on the Cleanse and feel better again, we marvelled at our enthusiasm. Our baggy eyes disappeared in three days. We looked and felt good again. Our energy returned along with our increasing love and gratitude for each other and God. In fact, almost every one of the symptoms we had developed disappeared within three days of cleansing.

A few days later we tried it again and ate cooked foods for another four days. This time we even had chocolates and pizza (we still refused to eat meat). The same symptoms of ill-health and lifelessness returned gradually. It was during this time that we truly embraced the raw food diet with the fervor of religious converts. We have developed an appreciation for God's raw, fresh foods that bring joy just to look at them in their lovely, pure simplicity. Eating God's untampered fresh foods brings greater life and energy into us instead of depleting us. It makes us feel good, the breath is fresher after eating it, the mental capacity is increased and uplifted and our love and joy towards all life is accelerated in its expansion. Blessed is the life that grows and provides real food and blessed are those who eat it in its raw and fresh state!

Our earnestness and zeal to conquer all desire for non-foods still remains. We know, so help us God, that all such lower desires will one day be mere fading memories, as we go forward on the path to complete purification of the physical structure.

How to Combat the Effects of the Occasional "Pig-Out"

If you have been working on cleaning yourself out but have the occasional splurge or "pig-out" (as the popular and accurate saying goes) you may experience regrets at what your body is going to have to go through. You may want to eliminate the effects of the "pig-out" as rapidly as possible. Here is what you can do:

1) take one heaping teaspoon of papaya powder (I use this when I eat anything other than fruit)
2) take 3 - 4 "Chomper"
3) drink lots of water
4) take as much cayenne as you can stand
5) take an enema before bed and one in the morning
6) take a psyllium shake when you get up in the morning

By noon the next day, everything will be okay again. Once, during our four-day experiment, we ate in what appeared to be one of the nicest restaurants in Klamath Falls, Oregon. We had good 'ole pancakes and omelettes (which we hadn't had in ages). The pancakes tasted so bad that I could only eat one of them. The omelette had a piece of ham in it, which to me rank the highest in levels of repulsiveness. There was some chile on it with meat. I picked it out the best I could and ate it. Y-U-K! It was the worst omelette ever. This was the ideal eating experience, we decided, to destroy all desire for cooked foods. We laughed all the way through breakfast. About one-half hour later I decided it had to go. We stopped the car. I put about four squirts of super-powerful lobelia extract (that's two-and-a-half times the dose required to induce vomiting) in water. I drank it down. Then I thought about what I had just eaten and took two more eye dropper shots, undiluted, straight into the mouth. Nothing happened. I couldn't believe it. I did it all over again. I used almost half an ounce of the lobelia extract. Believe me, that's enough to make a rhinoceros upchuck his cookies. Either it was just plain karma, or else we can assume that the cleaner the body becomes, the less effective lobelia is in it emetic effects. Even though I never did vomit, the lobelia did make me feel enormously better. A half-hour or so later we both took the psyllium shake using a good fluid ounce of hydrated bentonite and felt good the rest of the day.

If there's anything we have learned, it's that it is not beneficial to force yourself to eat any certain way for long periods of time. Give up things gradually. If you have a strong desire for perfect health you eventually lose the desires for non-foods when your body is ready to let go of them. I do not mean to imply that you should not set goals or give your human a good nudge in the right direction once in a while. But don't impose a lofty goal upon yourself, setting yourself up for failure and disappointment before you are really ready to embrace your noble effort and take it to the limit. Ask God to help you–that's the only way it can work. The human, of its puny self, is nothing. Read inspiring books about raw food diets. If you don't know of any, write to me and I will be happy to provide a list.

Secrets of Super Health

Keep in mind that fruit is the natural food for a clean, healthy body because it has the highest vibratory frequency of all foods. It is this higher vibratory level that allows man to tune into his true nature and his relationship with God. It has been said that God works for man, through man, as man, *when man is pure*. "Only the pure shall see God," warns the Bible. Granted, we must cleanse and purify our minds, emotions and actions—these, in fact, are more important to cleanse than the body. But many have found that in order to do that they must first cleanse the physical structure, for the condition of the physical structure affects the mind and the emotions (and vice versa). At the risk of being redundant, I will now repeat the following, which explains the state of man and his ability to raise himself. Now follow this closely:

- the cell structure, including the mucoid fecal structure, constantly radiates consciousness, just as everything does to some degree; it emits a vibratory frequency which reflects the thoughts and feelings we were experiencing at the time we ingested the substance which contributed to the creation of those cells

- when the mucoid layers break up and are pulled from the intestinal wall, this consciousness surfaces and can exert a great influence upon one; when that substance is evacuated it and its inherent consciousness no longer have an effect

- therefore, after the mucoid layers are thoroughly removed, it is much easier to eliminate and control desires, appetites and bad habits as well as negative thoughts and emotions

- cleansing the intestinal tract and eventually the whole cell structure opens wide the door to peace, harmony and happiness in the emotional world

- certain foods—those of the highest vibratory level should be eaten to maintain that purity of mind and body and those foods of a lower vibratory level (such as meat) should be avoided to shut the door to unwanted vibratory feelings (such as hate and anger); then the cell structure can eliminate every negative thought, feeling, habit or attitude once and for all

One secret to super health is to so cleanse the entire intestinal tract that one can live an energetic, happy life sustained by raw fruit alone (or Light alone—''breatharians'' actually do exist). This may include sprouted seeds and nuts. Before reaching that point, try a diet of raw fruits and raw vegetables when you're ready. Before attaining that goal, eat mostly raw fruits and vegetables (salads) with occasional lightly-steamed or cooked food to control cleansing reactions. During this stage, a baked potato or some steamed vegetables now and then are fine. One should cleanse or fast periodically, but especially during this period.

Before reaching that state of purity in your diet, all of the above-mentioned foods are appropriate as well as the occasional grains and squashes. Dr. Jensen advocates the use of these four grains only: millet, rye, yellow cornmeal and brown rice. They should be whole and natural. Sprouted grains and seeds are considered vegetables and are both good and alive. Any foods other than those just mentioned, will actually undermine your efforts and lead you backward. However, they can sometimes prove useful when controlling cleansing reactions.

Why Raw Foods Are the Perfect Food

Raw foods are the perfect food for man and can bring him exceptional health. They keep the body clean and congestion-free. Only raw foods have life force and enzymes, which are far more important to your health than vitamins, minerals and amino acids. Vitamins, minerals and amino acids can keep you alive, but life force and enzymes will keep you *vibrantly* alive. You can eat foods without life force or enzymes and still get minerals and proteins, but you cannot eat foods with life force and enzymes and not also get vitamins, minerals and proteins.

Alexis Carrel of the Rockefeller Institute and recipient of the Nobel Prize *was able to keep tissue cells alive indefinitely* by nutritious feedings and by washing away tissue excretions. The cells grew and thrived as long as evacuations were removed. Unsanitary conditions resulted in lower vitality, deterioration and death. He kept a chicken heart alive for 29 years until someone failed to cleanse its excretions!

The same holds true in the human body. If not kept clean inside, congestion occurs, the blood becomes impure and the result is lowered vitality, disease and a broken-down immune system which eventually leads to so-called death. How many times have you marvelled at the seemingly endless energy of the young child? Before the body is congested, when it is in its pure state, it is wonderfully alive, vibrant and bursting with energy. Congestion, which generally begins in the intestines, is really the number one killer in the world. Without congestion, the cells easily repair themselves. (Carrell believed that the cell was, therefore, immortal.) Congestion starves the cells of needed nutrients and oxygen. Dr. West claims one cannot die without congestion. The body is not only capable of repairing itself, but what's more it never stops trying! All we have to do is get out of its way. Most people know that if you put sugar into the gas tank, it clogs up the engine and the car stops running. Eating cooked and processed foods are like putting slime and glue into the body. No wonder the body wears out—it's been forced to work a few too many overtime hours!

So, the key is to eat foods that keep the body congestion-free. And that means raw fruits and raw vegetables. Moses lived 120 years. Methuselah lived over 900 years. Who knows how long we would live if we cleansed ourselves and ate raw foods? They are absolutely teeming with life force and enzymes.

Life Force

Life force is the most powerful and effective contributor toward good health there is. It is the source of energy and nerve power. It gives life to our cells and to the enzymes in our body.

Every atom of our bodies is filled with electricity or life force to some degree. These atoms are composed of electrons and protons, which are negatively and positively charged particles. The greater the force, charge or voltage of each atom, the more power it can generate to feed the life of each cell. The cell itself can be so charged with life force that it can become radiant light. It is the light that repels disease. Light is life. It is energy in its purest form. The greater the power flowing, the more one is able to think clearly and accurately. When this energy flows in full force through the nerve channels and emotional body, it is easier to remain positive in the feelings. Charismatic qualities of happiness and joy surface more readily. The mind and heart are naturally drawn to higher things. One is inclined to express love and kindness more freely and seldom tires at work or play. And when this life force flows through every cell of the body, we ward off disease, handle stress effectively, stay healthy longer and ultimately slow down the aging process.

The life force of the body is not dissipated or destroyed by over-exertion (for exercise eliminates toxins and hard breathing helps draw the life force back in). It is dissipated or destroyed by drugs, sex, negative emotions and dead foods. Foods that have been cooked, frozen, canned or processed have had the life force removed. Each time these dead or devitalized foods are consumed we are, in effect, "killing off" our energy, our aliveness, our health. And the process of aging speeds up. A good illustration follows: When one fully-charged 12-volt battery is hooked up to a dead 12-volt battery, the dead battery will draw from the charged battery until the median level is reached. The fully-charged battery becomes considerably drained—in fact, it is drained to half its original force.

And so it goes when eating dead foods. A portion of our life force is drained from our electrical reserves (located in the spine and in each atom) to feed the devitalized foods. On the other hand, eating raw foods help build the life force, adding zest and energy while keeping the body free from congestion. Eating raw food is like eating fully-charged battery cells.

Once we have eliminated all congestion from the body along with the congestion of negative thoughts and feelings, the life force connection with God and the solar system may flow in unlimited power through the other centers (which are now sealed) of the body. Who knows the potential in this? Only those who have attained this exalted state know and they are the legends of mankind's history. Ponder the words of Jesus: "All the things I have done you can also do and even greater things shall you do."

Enzymes

Raw foods are full of enzymes. Cooked and processed foods have none. Enzymes play a vital part in the digestion of our foods, in fighting disease and in breaking down foreign matter. With the decrease of enzymes, a process of internal decay rapidly develops, creating mounting problems in the body which can even be transmitted, through DNA, to one's future children.

Enzymes are essential in maintaining internal cleanliness, not to mention health, youth and strength. They are far more important than any other nutrient. Proteins cannot be utilized without enzymes, nor can vitamins and minerals. Enzymes are destroyed after use and must be constantly replaced. Cooked foods draw from the enzyme reserves, depleting the body's precious ''labor-force.'' Life force is the central core of each enzyme. Enzymes are the vehicles through which life force works to make things happen. Vitamins, minerals, proteins and body chemicals depend on enzymes to do all the work. Enzymes are the activity of life.

According to Dr. Edward Howell (who is probably the world's authority on enzymes) *each person is given a limited supply of body-enzyme energy at birth.* The faster we use up our enzyme supply, the shorter our life span, the weaker our immune system and the more dis-eased the body. As he puts it ''The habit of cooking our food and eating it processed with chemicals and the use of alcohol, drugs and junk food all draw out tremendous quantities of enzymes from our limited supply.'' He also says that colds, flu and other sickness deplete the supply.

Dr. Howell exposes the unsuccessful attempts of modern medicine to heal disease and its failure to attack the root of the problem. He says that many, if not all, degenerative diseases from which humans suffer and die are caused by excessive use of enzyme-deficient cooked and processed foods. This is one of the many reasons that herbs cure and drugs do not. Drugs have no life—no enzymes. But herbs do. By 1968 science had identified 1300 enzymes. There are three classes of enzymes—digestive enzymes which digest our food, food enzymes which are abundant in raw foods and metabolic enzymes. Food enzymes supply many of the digestive enzymes which the body would have to supply from its limited reserves if one ate cooked food. When we have lived for many years on cooked foods we can easily have depleted our digestive enzymes. When this happens our digestive system will withdraw from our metabolic enzyme reserves to aid in digestion. A shortage of metabolic enzymes, which the body uses to function, can cause serious malfunctions of the organs, glands, nerves, etc. As the metabolic enzymes are depleted to a certain point, the body begins to deteriorate. Science does not know how to replenish metabolic enzymes. A few digestive enzyme supplements are now available, but not metabolic enzymes. We believe there is a way to replenish these metabolic enzymes and have friends who have succeeded in doing this. Since we are still in the process of trying to prove it on ourselves, we feel we must wait to talk about it. Hopefully, we will publish our next book *Cleanse & Purify Thyself—Book II*. Maybe then we will be able to share what we know about complete renewal of the mental, emotional and physical structures.

Heating food over 116-120 degrees destroys all food enzymes (and vitamins) and forces the body to deplete itself. This causes enlargening of the digestive organs, especially the pancreas. Hot foods and hot drinks will injure the enzymes in the stomach.

Enzymes are the active ingredients that cure disease. They are the central core of the immune system and necessary for the maintenance of health. It is the enzymatic activity that makes your brain function and your memory work. It is what keeps your body alive. So, for a longer, healthier and happier life one should eat less and eat only raw foods. The words of Jesus Christ:

"So eat always from the table of God: the fruits of the trees, the grain and grasses of the field, the milk of beasts, and the honey of bees. For everything beyond these is of Satan, and leads by the way of sins and of diseases unto death. But the foods which you eat from the abundant table of God give strength and youth to your body, and you will never see disease. For the table of God fed Methuselah of old, and I tell you truly, if you live even as he lived, then will the God of the living give you also long life upon the earth as was his.

"For I tell you truly, the God of the living is richer than all the rich of the earth, and his abundant table is richer than the richest table of feasting of all the rich upon the earth. Eat, therefore, all your life at the table of our Earthly Mother, and you will never see want. And when you eat at her table, eat all things even as they are found on the table of the Earthly Mother. Cook not, neither mix all things one with another, lest your bowels become as steaming bogs. For I tell you truly, this is abominable in the eyes of the Lord.

"And be not like the greedy servant, who always ate up, at the table of his lord, the portions of others. And he devoured everything himself, and mixed all together in his gluttony. And seeing that, his lord was wroth with him, and drove him from the table. And when all had ended their meal, he mixed together all that remained upon the table, and called the greedy servant to him and said: 'Take and eat all this with the swine, for your place is with them, and not at my table.'

"Take heed, therefore, and defile not with all kinds of abominations the temple of your bodies. Be content with two or three sorts of food, which you will find always upon the table of our Earthly Mother. And desire not to devour all things which you see around you. For I tell you truly, if you mix together all sorts of food in your body, then the peace of your body will cease, and endless war will rage in you. And it will be blotted out even as homes and kingdoms divided against themselves work their own destruction. For your God is the God of peace, and does never help division. Arouse not, therefore, against you the wrath of God, lest he drive you from his table, and lest you be compelled to go to the table of Satan, where the fire of sins, diseases, and death will corrupt your body.

"And when you eat, never eat unto fulness. Flee the temptations of Satan, and listen to the voice of God's angels. For Satan and his power tempt you always to eat more and more. But live by the spirit, and resist the desires of the body. And your fasting is always pleasing in the eyes of the angels of God. So give heed to how much you have eaten when your body is sated, and always eat less by a third. Let the weight of your daily food be not less than a mina, but mark that it go not beyond two. Then will the angels of God serve you always, and you will never fall into the bondage of Satan and of his diseases. Trouble not the work of the angels in your body by eating often. For I tell you truly, he who eats more than twice in the day does in him the work of Satan. And the angels of God leave his body, and soon Satan will take possession of it. Eat only when the sun is highest in the heavens, and again when it is set. And you will never see disease, for such finds favor in the eyes of the Lord. And if you will that the angels of God rejoice in your body, and that Satan shun you afar, then sit but once in the day at the table of God. And then your days will be long upon the earth, for this is pleasing in the eyes of the Lord. Eat always when the the table of God is served before you, and eat always of that which you find upon the table of God. For I tell you truly, God knows well what your body needs, and when it needs."

(*The Gospel of Jesus Christ* by the Disciple John)

Healthy Bacteria

A healthy, "friendly" intestinal bacteria is essential to good health. Most raw foods, especially those with chlorophyll, feed the friendly bacteria. Cooked and processed foods feed the harmful bacteria. The friendly bacteria is needed to:

- reduce cholesterol in the blood
- produce certain necessary digestive enzymes
- control the pH factor or acidity-alkaline levels in the intestines
- reduce unhealthy bacteria in the intestinal tract
- reduce high blood pressure
- detoxify poisonous material in the diet
- strengthen the immune system
- assist in elimination of ailments such as colon irritation, constipation, diarrhea and acne
- manufacture and assimilate B-complex (which includes niacin, biotin, folic acid, riboflavin and B-12)
- helps digest proteins, carbohydrates and fats

- produces natural anti-bacterial agents (antibiotics) which inhibit 23 known pathogens
- produces cancer or tumor suppressing compounds
- detoxifies hazardous chemicals added to foods, such as nitrates
- increases calcium assimilation
- helps eliminate bad breath and gas
- retards yeast infections
- helps alleviate anxiety and stress
- retards proliferation of vaginitis, flus or herpes

It's interesting to me that opponents to vegetarianism insist that if one doesn't eat meat he has no source of vitamin B-12 and is undernourished. That theory is rather upside-down. Those who eat meat destroy the B-12 as soon as they cook it. Also, meat eaters generally have a very poor intestinal flora (little or no friendly bacteria) and are therefore unable to produce or assimilate B-12 properly. Vegetarians who have a healthy intestinal flora are able to produce it.

Here is a list of the most dangerous enemies of the friendly bacteria, in order of importance to be avoided:

- *drugs*—especially antiobiotics, as one dose can eliminate it all
- *alcohol*—it destroys enzymes and lacto bacteria, not to mention actual cells (particularly brain cells)
- *coffee*—each cup can destroy 20% of the friendly bacteria
- *meat*—it feeds the bacillus coli (harmful bacteria) which in turn destroy the good bacteria (yes, the body is a living episode of "Star Wars!")
- *bread*—especially white flour or any wheat bread that was baked in an oven
- *sugar*—yes, that includes most breakfast cereals, chocolate, cakes, pies, cookies, ice cream, pop, etc.
- *fried foods*—e.g. potato chips, fries and anything fried in oil

86

Because good health depends on having a balanced intestinal flora, there are many who constantly try to implant the healthy bacteria by taking acidophilus in its various forms. They generally fail in their efforts for one of two reasons: 1) successful implantation cannot occur until the intestines are cleaned out since harmful bacteria will always overrun the friendly bacteria before it can get a stronghold; and 2) acidophilus will not implant properly in humans. It seems that lacto bifidus and streptococcus will, which is why I recommend them in the "Clean-Me-Out Program". The problem is that most lacto acidophilus on the market is derived from a strain of animal bacteria (from cow's milk). Although it may assist human digestion because of its similarity to the human lacto bacteria, it must be constantly fed or replenished because it is not an exact duplicate of the human strain required and dies out easily (maybe because we don't eat the same things a cow does).

The lacto bifidus, on the other hand, is a strain of bacteria which is derived from human mother's milk. At birth, the infant who is breast-fed thus receives an immediate implant of friendly bacteria. That is why Nature designed mothers to breast feed their babies and why children who are not nursed are said to have more physical and emotional problems.

After cleansing the complete intestinal tract, implanting the friendly bacteria for a healthy intestinal flora and eating raw foods, you will be well on your way to a healthy, happy life!

9

THE EXPERIENCE IN NAPEEQUA

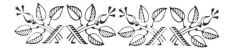

August, 1987, White Crow and I hiked about eight miles over Little Giant Pass (elev. 6400) into the Napeequa Valley of the North Cascades. This is one of the most secluded and rugged mountain valleys in the continental United States. First we waded through the Chiwawa River. Then we hiked on an old, delapidated trail which winds up through steep, rugged brush and rocks until it breaks into high, mountain meadows that stretch for miles on end. The first day we hiked until dark, which brought us past some rocky cliffs where the year before we had seen a bear and her cub. Then we broke into the meadows. Here we ate a few peaches and nectarines which were to be our last meal for six days. The purpose of this trip was to fast, drinking only water.

The next morning we hiked over the pass and down into one of the most scenic crops of mountains on the planet Earth. By the time we came to the river in the bottom of the Valley, we were already feeling the effects of the fast, for we had been living on raw fruits with occasional salads for several months. We didn't realize that our bodies were already cleansing at high speed. When we started this fast we, therefore, went into a maximum-cleansing mode.

We felt terrible. We set up the tent and took a cold bath in the river which was fed by several glaciers several miles upstream. It was cold, but the effect was marvelous. Three days passed. We were saved by those cold baths. We felt worse on this fast than any other fast or cleanse we'd ever been on. But we wanted to be rid of all toxins and poisons. We had developed a driving compulsion to be totally pure. Not only had we been working on the physical structure but we had been striving to purify every thought, feeling, appetite and desire. Much progress had been made and we hoped that a high level of purification would be attained with this fast.

The evening of the third day, I had just finished reading the book *The Gospel of Peace of Jesus Christ* by the disciple John. We crawled into our sleeping bags, hoping that we would sleep through until noon the next day.

My thoughts turned to my beloved wife. I let my thoughts drift with her. We were walking through beautiful, landscaped gardens, up a walkway to a pure, white temple. We were all dressed in white. We were prepared to enter the temple when an elderly couple approached. I recognized them. They had just been on the intestinal cleanse; their faces glowed with health, light shining in their eyes which were full of appreciation for the cleansing that had helped them so much. As I looked at their beaming faces, my love went forth with great intensity. I went up to them and put my arms around them. I was filled with a tremendous sense of appreciation for their willingness to purify themselves.

Tears of joy and love gathered and increased, until I felt embarrassed to show them; I turned to my wife and went to her. Another wave of even more intense love came. We walked to the trees and, again, a flood of love flowed through me, this time so powerfully that I awoke from my reverie. When the next wave came, I realized that my body was not pure enough to handle this much love for long. I positively knew that it would actually disintegrate if I felt this overwhelmingly powerful love much longer. As I enjoyed this immeasurable love and happiness, tears continued to flow and dampen my sleeping bag. I realized that I was having a profound Divine experience.

I opened my eyes. To my utter joy I saw right through the tent and there above me stood a beautiful and glorious Divine Being. Words cannot describe Her. Surrounded with an aura of light so bright that I could scarcely see the image within, she had lovely golden hair which fell below her shoulders and large, bright eyes filled with divine love, wisdom and power. She stood just a few feet above the tent. Millions of tiny, quarter-inch light rays rippled in various colors—blue, gold, pink, green, violet and white—and flowed gently at a 45-degree angle from Her into the earth.

Then Her most loving, sweet voice spoke these words: *"Blessed are you for your willingness to purify yourself; you shall be rewarded openly!"* Instantly I was filled with information I had not had a few seconds before. With absolute certainty I knew exactly what she meant. Anyone and everyone who willingly purified themselves—not only physically, but also mentally, emotionally, spiritually and completely—would receive rewards beyond their fondest dreams. Not only that, but this purification is a guaranteed entrance into what is called Heaven, for only those may enter therein who have first purified themselves. And those who are willing to do so shall have the help of God's mightiest messengers and, if necessary, legions of angelic beings. All must someday do this and the sooner, the better. For only the "pure shall see God" and only the pure may enter the gates of Heaven. This must be accomplished before one meets death.

This is the secret of secrets—even though it has already been proclaimed with clarity and practicality. It is in direct conflict with man's lusts, appetites and desires. The first offers divine benefits while the latter, only satanic pain.

I listened to Her words of wisdom and was then allowed to ask questions. My first question: "Were the words written in *The Gospel of Peace of Jesus Christ* by the disciple John the actual words of Jesus?" Her answer: "With the exception of a few translation errors, those words are the words of Jesus, and are true."

About then I jabbed White Crow with my elbow. He awoke. I found myself almost unable to talk. "Joseph," I said (his real name) "look above the tent! What do you see?" He saw Her. Blessed are we both. She asked me to include this experience in the next publication of my book. For about 30 more minutes we talked and for those 30 minutes we were filled with an essence of such love that made all things on earth seem small and insignificant in comparison. The only thing that seemed to matter on this level of existence was that which could assist us in permanently reaching this state of transcendent love and peace.

It was made crystal clear that all the studies and learning one could do amounted to nothing when compared to the need to purify the mind, feeling, habits and bodies. It is only through purification that one may obtain divine wisdom, love and power. It is only through purification that one can find entrance to the world of Heaven without passing through the change called death. All these things are possible for mortal man when he purifies. The full power of Christ can only function in a pure temple. The full power of Christ would disintegrate an impure body. Those millions—no, billions of mortal men expecting to find heaven upon death are in for a rude awakening. Jesus said, "Ye must be perfect *before* you enter the kingdom of heaven." Contrary to popular Christian belief, He meant exactly what He said.

Do not misunderstand this experience in Napeequa. It did not come about just because we had been physically cleansing our bodies. That was an important step. But even more important than that was how we had been cleansing the mind, feelings and spirit. Almost every imperfect thought, feeling, habit and negative experience of the past had been in the process of being brought forth and consumed.

There is a possibility that *Cleanse and Purify Thyself—Book II* will be published. This will reveal our experiences in eliminating the mental, emotional and etheric accumulations in our worlds that are less than perfect. All this began in the summer of 1987. We are still in this process of complete purification, but I can promise one thing: this return journey to God through complete purification has been unusual, enlightening and uplifting beyond our every expectation.

10

QUESTIONS AND ANSWERS

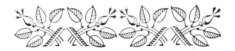

This section is devoted to answering the many questions that people have asked over the years.

Q—I am only 5 feet 5 and weigh 227 pounds. I lost almost 20 pounds while on the Cleanse, but now I am gaining weight again. What is wrong?

A—I have found that most people who are over-weight eat far too much acid food. We cannot continue eating acid foods and expect to be healthy. So far, in my experience, all obese people who have come to me and gone on an alkaline diet, have lost weight without starving themselves. In fact, they can eat all they want and still have success, but they must eat the right foods. However, there can be other factors such as the thyroid. When people have tried everything and nothing works for long, they need to look deep within themselves, root out the old consciousness, and replace it with a new image.

Q—I was on my second day of the Phase I Cleanse and followed the directions to the letter. I felt pain in my lower stomach. It continued to get worse and by the third day I had to stop the Cleanse, for the nausea and pain had become unbearable. I had passed a lot of the mucoid fecal matter, so I know that it is in there. I want to keep cleansing. What should I do?

A—You did the right thing by stopping the Cleanse. Having seen the iris of your eyes and knowing what you just went through, I would say you have some serious parasite activity. You're fortunate to have discovered it at such a young age. I am actually a little surprised, because your eyes indicated that you are far above average in your health, in your overall constitution and internal body cleanliness. You have no history of colitis or stomach problems. You followed the directions perfectly and had good elimination. People who have pain and nausea while on the Cleanse almost certainly have serious parasite infestation. Now there are three things one can do about it: 1) You could go back on the Cleanse and let it pull them out. However, the little buggers will fight you all the way. 2) You could take parasite vermifuge herbs while on the Cleanse and, hopefully, before the first day is over you could wipe out enough of them to keep them from causing you pain anymore. 3) You could stay off the Cleanse while you went on a parasite program for a week or two (eating while on it) and wait another two weeks and do it again to get the littles ones that would then be hatching from the eggs. Remember, *you won't be rid of all your worms until you've cleaned out the mucoid layers they hide in.* But at least you can wipe out enough of them to keep them from bothering you.

Q—I take that "Psyllium Shake" and my stomach hurts!

A—In all the years I've been doing this in one form or another and watching others do it, I have known this to happen only five times. One person was taking too much psyllium, two had worms and the remaining two were White Crow and myself. Here's what happened to us: After reaching a state of health beyond anything I'd ever known, I was on my way to the North Cascades from California with White Crow. It was 2:00 am when we reached Eugene, Oregon. We needed some rest. Since we prefer the stars to motels, we settled our sleeping bags on some grass about 200 yards from a sheriff training area. Just at the crack of dawn, helicopters began flying low, passing over us. They continued for a couple of hours. We figured they were on some kind of maneuvers, since we were so close to the training area. As we were packing up to leave around 8:00 am, a woman came over to our car and warned us that we had probably just been sprayed with the Gypsy Moth BT chemical. Bless her heart! She gave us some information on it and we looked for clues—no unusual substance on the car or our sleeping bags; no odd smells. We felt great. About 24 hours later we were vomiting. Our stomachs swelled up; we kept burping up a horrible chemical stench; we felt spacey and disoriented; we later developed rashes which turned into oozing, itching welts, lost our coordination, had uncontrollable appetites for food we shouldn't eat and lost enough of our mental capacities to not even think how we could heal ourselves. We were unbelievably miserable! We stayed at my mother's in Seattle for one week until we got a little stronger. Then we headed for the mountains and tried to heal our sores. Using clay, we got rid of the rash in less than a week. The bloated stomach and burping lasted another three weeks. We finished our herb hunts and headed back to California.

One night, south of Salem, we camped on a vacant lot. It was late. We didn't think that BT sprays could be there because we were in a different county. Twenty-four hours later, it happened again. Bloated stomachs and the works. Crow had it even worse. He had slept on the grass; I had slept on a tarp. We tried fasting and it made us deathly sick. My toe nails turned black. My front tooth turned black, then it became brittle and chipped. Finally, the body stored away the sprays. I got better, but not back to normal. I went on the Cleanse, which is what I should have done in the first place. I began to have pains in my stomach. Why? Because the body began to release the sprays it had conscientiously stored in a cyst-like case. It wouldn't let it go through my system and destroy me. The body is fantastic! Then the psyllium shake began to extract the BT. I immediately felt better, so I increased the bentonite quite a bit. POW! I was hurtin'! Because the pain was so great I stayed flat on my stomach. Each time I vomited I smelled those chemicals. Finally, I vomited a glob of white slime and—bingo!—it was over. I started feeling great again. White Crow had the exact same experience the next time he went on the Cleanse. After passing a huge, white, slimy fuzzball he sure felt better. No more stomach pains! (Note: The Gypsy Moth BT spray is said to be non-toxic to humans, believe it or not. If ever you have the opportunity to give your input at the public hearings, I would urge you to do so. There is an untold, heavy toll for the spraying of toxic chemicals on public lands.)

Q—Will I lose much weight while on the "Clean-Me-Out Program?"

A—Obese people can lose quite a lot of weight while on the Program. Thin people will gain whatever they lose about two or three days after finishing the Cleanse (minus the weight of whatever mucoid layers they passed). Sometimes thin people will continue to put on weight after cleansing.

Q—Is it okay to take a colema or colonic?

A—If it works for you, go ahead. Both are good methods for those who are able to get the liquid to flow all the way to the ileocecal while resting on the back. I would recommend either over the enema. Colonics are rather expensive. But while on the Cleanse, if you can afford it, take them. Some claim that colemas make the bowels stronger. Actually the main difference between the colema or colonic and the enema is that they use more water and it's easier to massage the abdomen while on the back. In the "Clean-Me-Out Program" it's the "Chomper" that makes the bowels stronger. The herbs in that formula not only clean the intestinal wall but stimulate and nourish it. Cold-water enemas will also strengthen the bowels.

Q—Can the enema water flow into the small intestine?

A—If your ileocecal valve somehow was stuck open, it could. But that is a rare malfunction of the body and nothing would be better for that condition than the Cleanse.

Q—Will the "Clean-Me-Out Program" remove diverticuli?

A—It can, eventually, as long as proper eating habits, exercise, enemas and herbs are consistently used.

Q—I feel sick to my stomach! I don't want to do this anymore!

A—The only two reasons you have nausea are 1) because of the toxins you put in there or 2) because the parasites in your stomach are mighty upset that you are disturbing them. If it's toxins, you'll have to tough it out if you want to get them out of there and improve your health. That will take dedication and determination. As you may have gathered, purification is not for the average individual. If it's due to parasites, refer to the second question in this chapter. No matter which one is the cause, it wouldn't hurt to take an enema if you're feeling nauseated. It may do a world of good.

Q—I don't want to take enemas anymore. They make me feel weak.

A—That happened to me a couple of times. Again, it's because of the toxins. Remember, sometimes things must get stirred up before they can be removed. Stick it out, remove the toxins quickly with an enema and you'll perk up for sure.

Q—Can I take the lacto bifidus while on the Cleanse?

A—No. The psyllium and bentonite would absorb it before it had any effect. Wait until after the Cleanse.

Q—I'm on my second day and feeling very tired. In fact, I'd just like to stay in bed. What will I be like in seven days?

A—Your weakness is probably due to the amount of toxic substances you are eliminating. Generally, people who are weak on the second and third days perk up by the fourth. Until then, go ahead and get the rest your body wants. If weakness persists, consider switching over to *Phase II—Easy Does It* and eat one meal a day.

Q—Boy, do I have a lot of gas! What now?

A—When you have too much gas or have a headache or any other pains, take an enema.

Q—I guess I'm feeling okay on this Cleanse. But I feel a little sluggish.

A—Drink more liquids, take an enema and take chlorella.

Q—Rich, I think I've just lost part of my intestines. Maybe I'd better go to a doctor. You should see what just came out of me!

A—CONGRATULATIONS! You just passed a layer of hardened, mucoid fecal matter. When it first happened to me, I thought the very same thing.

Q—What's the big deal about what water I use in the enema? After all, it's just going in and coming right back out with all that garbage!

A—During your enema you will always absorb some of the liquid. Unless you live in a very pure environment, *beware of* chlorine and sodium fluoride in water. Sodium fluoride is a waste product from aluminum milling companies. By selling it for 1.5 cents a pound, they make $15,000,000 a year profit. The reason it managed to be sold in the first place is that it was known that in certain areas of the country where *calcium* fluoride was abundant in water, there was little tooth decay. Unfortunately, and evidently without complete investigation, the F.D.A. approved its use and into the water system of major American cities *sodium* (not calcium) fluoride went. Eventually the truth came out—the use of sodium fluoride in tap water led to a 50% increase of tooth decay, a 12% increase of Mongoloid children and a massive increase of Alzheimer's disease. Isn't the F.D.A. something? *Sodium fluoride is a deadly poison* that is used to kill rats by destroying the digestive system. Keep in mind that *sodium* fluoride and *calcium* fluoride are not at all the same thing. And anyone making decisions for the F.D.A. should know that.

Q—Should I continue to take my medication while on the "Clean-Me-Out Program?"

A—I really cannot advise you on that one. Use your own discretion or talk to your doctor about it. Read *World Without Cancer*, by Edward Griffin. Find out the facts about drugs.

Q—While on the Cleanse, I notice that I sometimes feel dizzy when I stand up.

A—This is a common occurrence. The stirred-up toxins are the cause. After cleansing the body of the toxins, the dizziness will go away.

Q—I have a weak heart. I notice that during this Cleanse it pounds a lot.

A—Supposedly I have a weak heart, too. In fact, I'm also supposed to have bad valves and an enlarged heart because of rheumatic fever. My heart used to pound while on the Cleanse occasionally. Releasing drugs and other toxins can make anyone's heart do that. But it doesn't happen to me anymore. If you get really concerned, take cayenne pepper in warm water. I have written an article about cayenne pepper (capsicum) and its benefits to the heart. It can stop a heart attack or stroke in 30 seconds when administered correctly. Write to the address on page 110 for more on cayenne.

Your question reminds me of my mother who is one of the neatest people you could ever meet; she gets straight A's in personality. She had always trusted the A.M.A.'s treat-the-symptom syndrome. Her faith in that area has dwindled to a low ebb, but only after watching her mother die a horrible, unnecessary, slow, painful death and having seen so many of friends and relatives suffer needlessly. She has always marvelled at the wonders of science—particularly medical science. When her hip started giving her trouble, she began to hope for a bionic hip. I did my best to try and convince her to try healing herself Nature's way—with herbs. My efforts were in vain. She eventually got her wish and had a bionic hip put in. She loved it! But after her operation she never could seem to enjoy her original active condition. Her heart was bothering her. She kept taking all of the wizard-like concoctions her doctor would give her, all to no avail. Finally, one day I left her just a few cayenne capsules saying, "Mother, it can't hurt you! It's just food. There's nothing better for your heart! Just take two and see what happens." She said, "Well, maybe" as I left.

The next day she was again very tired. She was just going to take a mid-morning nap on the couch. She went into the kitchen for one more thing and saw those cayenne capsules laying on the counter and decided to try one (even though I had told her to try two). She swallowed it down and went to get a book to read and headed for the couch. She started to lay down and suddenly stopped and said to herself "Wait a minute! I'm feeling pretty good!" Not only did she dispense with the nap, she ended up spending the whole day working in the yard and called to tell me to order her a large bottle of cayenne. She has been taking them ever since along with hawthorn and garlic and her health is getting stronger as she cleanses her bloodstream of free radicals and cholesterol. Remember, cayenne is loaded with vitamin A, C and potassium—the heart mineral.

Q—I'm pregnant and would like to start cleansing. Is it okay?

A—Though many pregnant women have successfully used the Clean-Me-Out Program with great success, I do feel that I should give advice in this area. Each situation is unique in itself. Each person must seek the advice within and make her own decision as to how she should conduct her life. Ideally, every woman should cleanse her body temple before becoming pregnant and then be sure to acquire the best of nutrition for herself and her new baby. My only suggestion is for the potential mother to drink at least one or two cups of Red Raspberry tea each day during pregnancy. Drinking this tea can solve many problems and make the entire pregnancy and delivery easy, enjoyable, and successful.

Q—I'm considering doing the Cleanse, but I don't know if it's for me. What if I get hungry?

A—You don't get hungry on this Cleanse. You can't. You'll be stuffed with herbs and liquids. But if you think you're hungry, drink diluted juice or herbal teas, or follow *Phase II—Easy Does It.*

Q—A doctor told me it wasn't necessary to replace the intestinal bacteria right after colon cleansing and that I could just wait a few months.

A—After cleansing, most bacteria have been removed (that's both friendly and harmful bacteria). The tendency for growth is predominantly toward the bacillus coli and other harmful bacteria. After the Cleanse, the implanting of lacto bifidus has the best opportunity ever to get its stronghold, since this is when the other bacteria are at their minimum. Once the lacto bifidus is well-established, it will fight off the bacillus coli that may attempt to establish itself.

Q—I've been told by my doctor that I have a spastic colon and that I'd better be careful with colon cleansing. What do you think?

A—I agree. Be careful. If I had your conditions (which could cause pain) I would cut down on the recommended dosages of psyllium. I would also use catnip tea enemas made with distilled water to relax the colon. I would be very generous with the catnip enema. Believe me, though, if I had a spastic colon I sure wouldn't hesitate to cleanse. I would do anything and everything I could to repair that area now and not wait until I felt worse.

Q—What about using bentonite in my enemas?

A—That would be an excellent way to absorb toxic substance. Clay, especially bentonite, is an excellent healer. It can be used for all sorts of things—sores, wounds, rashes, cysts and anything that has toxins which need to be drained. Bentonite comes in both powder and liquid form. Write to the address on page 110 for further information on the uses of bentonite.

Q—Is it true that lacto bacteria can be destroyed when you take a colonic?

A—Yes, if there is chlorine in the water. But chances are if you need a colonic, the lacto bacteria in your colon has already been overrun by the harmful bacteria.

Q—Do you recommend rejuvelac?

A—I have tried it without results. But, in all fairness, I did not give it much of a try. I plan to experiment with it again.

Q—My menstrual periods have changed since I've been cleansing. Is that normal?

A—Actually, that is common among women who cleanse. It changes as the body becomes cleaner. Contrary to popular belief, menstrual discharges are not natural to women. They're just a way the body has of cleansing itself of impurities. So, the purer a woman's body becomes, the less discharge there will be, until eventually there will be none at all. I have a friend in Wenatchee, Washington who, after one-and-a-half years on raw food followed by two-and-a-half years on fresh fruit, at last found she no longer had any menstrual discharge. People used to guess her to be 23 to 29 years old when she was 44!

Q—If I eat yogurt do I need the bifidus cultures you recommend for the Program?

A—Yogurt will not be able to replenish the intestines with the correct amounts of flora. Even if it did implant successfully, the eating of dairy products creates so much mucus and congestion in the body that it would be truly counter-productive. (One exception: if the yogurt was made fresh and raw from goat's milk it would probably be very good for you.)

Q—I've noticed that there are other psyllium products on the market that contain added enzymes, herbs, bentonite and acidophilus all in one container. Wouldn't it be a better way to go?

A—Not in my opinion. The herbs are taken separately from the psyllium and bentonite on the "Clean-Me-Out Program" for a definite reason. The herbs, which move out into the mucoid matter to break it up and feed the intestines, have the opposite effect of th⁻ psyllium and bentonite, which attract toxins, bacteria and debris froı the intestines. The psyllium and bentonite hold the harmful substanc in one mass until the body evacuates it. Any enzymes, herbs or friendly bacteria in the bulk mixtures you mention would never be released to do their job. Therefore, the substances in these mixtures are excellent by themselves, but ineffective when mixed together and taken all at once.

Q—What about using psyllium seeds instead of husks?

A—I wouldn't recommend it. The seeds, when wet, form a gel that has a different activity than the husks. This activity interferes with the bentonite and does not hold the mucoid layer as the psyllium husk powder can.

Q—Can I take montmorillonite instead of bentonite?

A—Montmorillonite is the active ingredient in bentonite. In other words, they are the same thing.

Q—Someone told me to drink carrot juice while on the Cleanse because it would help with the feeding and strengthening of the constructive mucous lining of the intestines.

A—If you wish to slow the cleansing down, go ahead. As far as carrot juice is concerned, it could only help the intestinal mucous lining if it could get through the mucoid layers. So drink this wonderful drink, but *after* cleansing.

Q—Is it okay for my children to go on the Cleanse?

A—You bet! Get them off to a great start. Why make them go through what most of us went through (and who knows what would have been ahead if we hadn't cleansed relatively early in life)? Children from five to ten years of age should have their dosages of bentonite and psyllium cut in about half. Regulate the "Chomper," too. And make certain they take their enemas twice a day.

Q—Will this "Clean-Me-Out Program" work if I continue to eat meat?

A—First of all, let me stress the importance of taking "Chomper" and "Herbal Nutrition" for at least a month before going on the Cleanse if you are a meat eater. Realize that your body is more toxic than that of the vegetarian and must be given a longer pre-cleanse preparation.

The "Clean-Me-Out Program" will remove the mucoid matter with you the same as it would with anyone. But you will just put it back into your body if you go back to your meat-eating habits after the Cleanse. You must seriously ask yourself: "what's more important to me, devouring animal cadavers or my health?" Once you have cleaned your body out you will find your desire for meat disappearing. I was once the biggest advocate for meat-eating you could find. I remember specifically telling my brother that he could be sure of two things: 1) I would never stop hunting, and 2) I would never stop eating meat. I thought that vegetarians were nuts and my body sure suffered for it. I was the one with oatmeal for brains! Thank God, I was wise enough to mend my ways. I learned to love animals and appreciate good health and not take it for granted.

Q—In the past, I've taken medicine with terrible side effects. Occasionally, I re-experience these side effects when I least expect it. Will cleansing help this?

A—Drugs can settle anywhere, including the intestines. They are like time bombs. Sometime, somewhere in the body, they may come loose and get reactivated. This can be very hard on the body, especially since it is most likely very different than it was when the drugs were ingested. It would be the part of wisdom, therefore, to cleanse because the psyllium and bentonite will absorb much of the toxic substance and you should not have to experience its maximum destructive potential as you might have otherwise. It came to pass recently that my wife and I were in Birmingham talking with a sweet lady suffering from Parkinson's Disease and diabetes. She expressed frustration and dissatisfaction with the effects of the drugs she had been taking as well as the numerous doctors she had gone to. She had recently spent $5,000 on tests which were to determine what was causing her so many problems. I reached into my pocket and pulled out my mini-flashlight and magnifying glass. I looked at the iris of her eyes. In less than five minutes I could tell not only what her problems were (and their stages of degeneration), but the cause of those problems. I could also tell her what she could do about them. It was so simple to do, and it didn't cost her a dime!

Oh, how many times do I hear the same old story—a trusting individual goes from doctor to doctor and pays and pays and pays, but only gets worse and worse and worse! When, oh when, will people learn? If something doesn't work, stop what you're doing and do something else. If a doctor has no history of healing a disease, why go to him? I would NEVER take my car in for a transmission repair if the mechanic had never been able to repair one before. We all have our choices—we can go God's way or man's way. We can trust Nature's herbs or man's drugs. Herbs cleanse, purify and heal. Drugs suppress, clog and destroy.

Q—Will the Cleanse help the immune system?

A—The body's natural immune system cannot be repaired in a toxic body. If your body is toxic, it is already overworked. Internal cleansing is a must. Also, use the following herbs: echinacea, capsicum, ginseng, dulse and alfalfa.

Q—Do you recommend the Cleanse for all diseases?

A—WARNING: Those with tuberculosis, cancer, emphysema, diabetes and other degenerative diseases should be assisted by expert health professionals who have a high success rate in those areas. Diabetics should consider fasting after receiving expert advice to do so.

But, to answer your question, if I were suffering from one of those diseases, I would most certainly cleanse. How do you think people get those diseases in the first place? Following *Phase II—Easy Does It* would be what I would do.

Q—I've heard skin brushing is a good way to cleanse. Do you agree?

A—Absolutely! Skin brushing is actually better than using soap. Soap will not clean your skin as well as skin brushing with a natural bristle brush will. (Avoid nylon brushes.) Soap removes only a small portion of the dead skin, while skin brushing removes all of the dead skin and dirt with it. Soap often clogs the skin's pores and inhibits its elimination. Skin brushing removes acids from the body and stimulates the skin by causing new blood to flow and circulate through this major elimination organ. Don't let your skin become lazy and overworked when just three-to-five minutes of skin brushing before your bath or shower will renew and strengthen it.

(It is best to brush the skin while it is dry, since it is said that brushing it while wet causes the skin to sag.)

Q—Do you recommend using digestive aids when I'm not on the Cleanse?

A—Until you become a fruitarian, I certainly do. There is one super digestive aid on the market now which not only heals the digestive tract, but help dissolve undigested protein which often tries to settle in the intestinal tract and make trouble. (Remember that undigested proteins are the number one favorite food of parasites and bacillus coli.) This product is called GREEN PAPAYA POWDER. Not only is it 100% pure, but it's 99.4% papaya. The rest of the contents are .4% guava and .2% lime. Produced by *Papaya Products of Hawaii*, it should be in your health food store. If not, it can also be ordered through mail order health food supplement distributors.

Green Papaya Powder contains a complex of enzymes that helps digest proteins, fats and carbohydrates. It's loaded with vitamin A, C, E and B factors. It is the highest source of papain you'll find, which is a superior aid to pepsin and pancreatin. We sprinkle it over our food (especially salads). You can feel it harmonizing the body. As White Crow says, "I don't like to be without it!"

Q—*Irradiated foods*—I've been hearing about them and they sound scary to me. Do you know anything about this?

A—Thanks for asking. Irradiation is a new, tremendously effective and diabolical method of preserving fresh fruits and vegetables which has recently gained nation-wide acceptance. It is extremely popular with the supermarkets because it will increase their profits, since their produce will now have a longer "shelf life".

Why is irradiation so bad? Because it destroys the enzymes in the food. This is what the process consists of: they put the food on pallets and drive them into huge vaults; then they seal the door and turn on the nuclear radiation. If a person were in the vault during this process, he would die instantly. All this just to make the fruits and vegetables last longer! The reason they do is because there is nothing else left alive in them to cause further ripening. Thus, even when individuals try to eat live foods they are eating dead foods!

At this rate, in about ten years the health of the American people will be at such a low ebb that frightening plagues or epidemics are likely to occur. This has already been expected among many health experts. With irradiated foods now in action, the time for plagues may come even sooner than predicted. When or if it does happen, we may thank the American Medical Association and its partner the Food and Drug Administration. They certainly have gone the extra mile to make America the sickest nation in the world. Some people may say we aren't the sickest nation—there are nations starving to death. Starvation is not necessarily a disease. But we're talking about degenerative diseases. Even among the starving nations, they have less heart and lung diseases, little cancer and little diabetes. We have no excuse to be sick. They do.

But the good thing about all this is that you don't have to be a part of it. Support your local health food stores which are trying to get you good, wholesome foods. Buy organically-grown produce. Even though it is more expensive it usually tastes better! And who knows what all those chemicals in and on the supermarket food will do to our bodies over long periods of time? The F.D.A. removes chemicals from the market many times a year because they are found to be harmful. Then it allows a new, harmful chemical to take its place, etc., etc., etc. This is similar to the habits of the A.M.A. with their involvement in the use of drugs. Constant replacement of harmful drugs with "new drugs" occurs. How many times have you heard your doctor say, "We have a new drug we're experimenting with." The only reason they are not using the last experimental drug is because it didn't work or was found to be harmful. So, now they are trying a new one . . . on who? Back in 1910, a man named Adolf Just wrote a book called *Return to Nature*. His success brought thousands of so-called incurables to him. Here is a quote from his book, concerning remedies:

> "All remedies that have not been taken from Nature, and are
> not in accordance with her, prove futile; no matter how often,
> apparently, they may have operated (seemingly) beneficially
> and effectively. There are too many deceptions here. The injury
> that inevitably accompanies all unnatural remedies, sooner or

later, always comes to the surface and causes them to disappear again, unfortunately only after much harm has been done. Such unnatural or not strictly natural remedies come and go, therefore, and will never find an abiding place of refuge.

"We see accordingly new remedies rising to the surface daily in medicine, only to disappear again as quickly as they came. Today carbolic acid, tomorrow palicylic acid, now antifebin, again Koch's lymph is the elixir upon which the safety and happiness of mankind is said to depend, until it has become clear that they work only harm and disaster. At present we calmly allow ourselves to be most seriously injured by remedies whose dangerous character can reveal itself only in the future."

Sound familiar?

Q—Everyone in my family has died of cancer and I have it, too. Doctors couldn't help them and they haven't helped me. I know that if I'm going to get well I have to find another way. Can you help me?

A—I would love to help you and I believe I could, but it's against the law for me to do it. It's something to think about, isn't it? It's against the law for those who know how to cure cancer to do it, but it's lawful for those who don't know how to treat it. In fact, in California it was against the law to treat cancer by any other method but surgery, drugs and radiation. Those methods have never eliminated the *cause* of cancer and yet no other method is allowed. Doesn't that boggle the mind? Do you realize what power the A.M.A. wields? One more thought: I have a document written by a doctor who investigated cancer statistics. He says that, on an average, *people who have terminal cancer live eight years longer if they never go to a medical doctor.* I wish everyone would read *Confessions of a Medical Heretic,* by Dr. Robert Mendelsohn as well as *World Without Cancer,* by Edward Griffin.

Fortunately, you still have the freedom to do to yourself whatever you want. In some states, however, you do not have the freedom to listen to whatever you want—i.e. someone whom you think can help you. A sinister influence was trying to make this happen in

California (as well as other states of the nation) with the introduction of the Dietitian's Monopoly Bill a few years ago.

If enacted, this bill would have made it a serious crime, punishable by heavy fines and imprisonment, for anyone who is not a licensed dietitian to give specific "nutritional counseling" to another person. It exempts medical doctors and a few other individuals. Spokespersons for the American Dietetic Association have made it clear that far from exempting those working in the health food industry—they intended to use the bill to silence, prosecute and imprison them. It condescendingly provided that those who are not licensed dietitians will not be prevented from furnishing "general" nutrition information. However, this "general" information can only be about "nutrition for healthy people." In a 300-word definition, the bill makes it a serious crime for a person who is not a licensed dietitian to provide "nutrition care," "nutrition services," "nutrition counseling," or "nutrition education." It is strongly supported by the American Dietetic Association (A.D.A.) and the American Medical Association (A.M.A.).

The American Heritage Dictionary defines "counsel" as: "an exchange of opinions and ideas." Therefore, the A.D.A. and the A.M.A. sought through A.B. 2369 to be given a monopoly over the exchanging of opinions and ideas about nutrition in California (and other states). A.B. 2369 conceded (on page one of the bill): "Existing law (already) makes it unlawful for a person to hold himself or herself out as a dietitian or registered unless he or she meets specified qualifications." This is as far as the law should go. There is a form letter that you can use to send to your assemblyperson which finishes as follows:

"I agree with the National Health Federation (N.H.F.), that given the deep hostility and intolerance exhibited by the A.D.A. against the millions of health minded Californians who happen to disagree with many of their rigid, narrow, and outdated ideas about diet and nutrition, that dietitians should not be licensed in California. I respectfully urge you, therefore, to kill—not amend—A.B. 2369. Thank you for preserving my health freedom."

This is an example of proposed laws that the N.H.F. uncovers so as to warn us of threats to our health freedoms. Their magazine, <u>Health Freedom News</u>, provides timely updates on many areas of health. If you would like information on how to subscribe, write NHF, Box 688, Monrovia, California 91016 or telephone (818) 357-2181.

To order the book Cleanse & Purify Thyself contact your local distributor or health food store or write to:

TRIUMPH BUSINESS
P.O. Box 1320
Mt. Shasta, California 96067

For information about ordering products for the

CLEAN-ME-OUT
PROGRAM

contact your local distributor or health food store or write to:

ARISE & SHINE
P.O. Box 901
Mt. Shasta, California 96067

12

BIBLIOGRAPHY AND SUGGESTED READING LIST

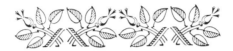

Dr. Baker and Elizabeth Baker. *The UNcook Book,* 1980. Drelwood Publications.

Dr. Banner, Donald. *Applied Iridology and Herbology,* 1982. Bi-World Publishers, Orem, Utah.

Cheadle and Levanthal. *Medical Parasitology,* 1985. F.A. Davis Company, Philadelphia, Pennsylvania.

Dr. Christopher, John R. *Dr. Christopher Talks on Rejuvenation Through Elimination,* 1976. Also, *Regenerative Diet,* 1982. Christopher Publications, Springville, Utah.

Dr. Dextreit, Raymond. *Our Earth, Our Cure,* 1974. Swan House Publishing Company, Brooklyn, N.Y.

Diamond, Harvey. *A Case Against Medicine,* 1979. Golden Glow Publishers, Santa Monica, California.

Disciple John. *The Gospel of Peace of Jesus Christ.* Also available under the title, *The Essene Gospel of Peace,* 1981. International Biogenic Society, Apartado #372, Cartago, Costa Rica, Central America.

Dufty, William. *Sugar Blues,* 1965. Nutri-Books Corporation, Box 5793, Denver, Colorado, 80217.

Ehret, Professor Arnold. *Mucusless Diet Healing System,* 1953. Also, *Rational Fasting,* 1965. Ehret Publishing Company, Los Angeles, California.

Fathman, George and Doris. *Live Foods—Nature's Perfect System of Human Nutrition.* Ehret Literature Publishing Company, Beaumont, California, 92223. (Includes 192 raw food recipes.)

Gray, Robert. *The Colon Health Handbook,* 1984. Rockridge Publishing Company, Oakland, California.

Griffin, Edward. *World Without Cancer.* Nutri-Books, Denver, Colorado.

Dr. Howell, Edward. *Enzyme Nutrition,* 1985. Avery Publishing Group, Inc., Wayne, New Jersey.

Hunter, Beatrice. *Consumer Beware! Your Food and What's Been Done to It.* Nutri-Books, Denver, Colorado.

Irons, V.E. *The Destruction of Your Own Natural Protective Mechanism.*

Dr. Jensen, Bernard. *Tissue Cleansing Through Bowel Management,* 1981. *Iridology: The Science and Practice of the Healing Arts, Volume II,* 1982. *Food Healing for Man.* Jensen Publishing Company, Escondido, California.

Kloss, Jethro. *Back to Eden,* 1975. Lifeline Books, Santa Barbara, California.

Dr. Mendelsohn, Robert. *Confessions of a Medical Heretic,* 1980. Warner Books, New York, New York.

Dr. Nolfi, Kirstine. *The Raw Food Treatment of Cancer and Other Diseases.* Leaves of Autumn Books, Payson, Arizona.

Parham, Barbara. *What's Wrong With Eating Meat?* Ananda Marga Publications, Denver, Colorado.

Ramacharaka, Yogi. *The Hindu Yogi Practical Water Cure,* 1935. The Yogo Publication Society, Chicago, Illinois.

BIBLIOGRAPHY & SUGGESTED READING

Sitt, Paul. *Fighting the Food Giants,* 1980. Nutri-Books, Denver, Colorado.

Tenney, Louise. *Today's Herbal Health,* 1983. Woodland Books, Provo, Utah.

UPDATES

CHECK-OFF LIST FOR EVERYONE

• **Before doing either Phase II or I, be sure to do the pH test and pass.** If you do not pass the pH tests, you can still do Phase III. But build up your electrolyte reserve before doing Phase II or I. See next section about pH.

• Every person reacts differently to every herb, food, treatment, etc. No one but your own special body knows for sure what it needs, so listen to it carefully. **Do not cleanse until you feel that it is really right for you.**

• Always do Phase III first, before doing any other phase. **It usually takes a minimum of one week before the herbs have prepared the mucoid plaque to be eliminated.** It is a waste of time to do Phase I without doing Phase III first. **THIS IS EXTREMELY IMPORTANT.** First time cleansers should do 4 weeks of Phase III before going into a deeper phase.

• If you begin to feel poorly after you have moved from Phase III into a deeper phase (Phase II or I), then go back to a milder phase. When people are extremely toxic, any kind of cleansing can cause cleansing reactions. **DO NOT ALLOW YOURSELF TO FEEL BAD.** It is not necessary to suffer. Do not try and be a hero by pushing yourself through toxic overloads. This could injure the liver or kidneys. Therefore, **it's very good to alternate with any of the three phases, as needed.**

• Whenever cleansing or fasting, a great deal of toxins and mucus can enter the blood stream. Because of this extra sludge in the blood, when you stand up it may take longer for oxygen to get into the brain. Therefore, **never stand up quickly when fasting or cleansing. Sit up first and then slowly stand up.** Some people have stood up too fast and have passed out. Don't let this happen to you.

• If your stomach is sensitive to the Chomper, you can separate them by five minutes. That is, take one (1) Chomper with one (1) Herbal

Nutrition, wait 5 minutes, then take one (1) of each again. Wait 5 minutes and repeat until you've taken the full amount. Also, ginger/ fennel tea will help settle the stomach.

• Remember that the Chomper has some laxative effects and the bentonite the opposite. So balance everything according to your own body.

• The intelligent use of Chomper and bentonite controls the consistency of the stool. It should be loose but not runny.

• If you get constipated, increase Chomper, or take an enema. If only 1 or 2 Chomper causes diarrhea, either increase bentonite in the shakes, or add Chomper Enhancer.

• If you have trouble getting the enema water to flow out of the bowels: 1. First try drinking about 16 ounces of water about 15 minutes before the enema. 2. If this doesn't work, then make a tea with wild cherry bark and add to the enema water. To make this tea, add 1 heaping teaspoon of wild cherry bark to a quart of water. Lightly simmer with lid on pot for 10 minutes. Strain and add to enema water, making a total of 4 to 6 quarts.

• Be sure to use pure powdered psyllium husks. Do not use psyllium seed powder; it will not work for the Cleanse. You can use whole or coarse psyllium husks, but you will need twice as much.

• When using this Cleanse, never use any psyllium containing any medicinal herbs such as cascara, goldenseal, etc. Medicinal herbs taken at the same time as psyllium, will completely disrupt the process. Never take bacteria along with psyllium shakes because the shakes will absorb most of the bacteria.

• If you are allergic to psyllium, use equal parts of psyllium husk powder, corn silk, and guar gum.

• Be sure to wait the full 1½ hours after all psyllium shakes before starting the herbs. You can take psyllium shakes 1 hour after taking the herbs to make up for lost time.

• Never use any kind of salt either orally or rectally when doing the

Cleanse. Some people have used salt water enemas or have taken salt water to cleanse their bowels. Absolutely nothing is more harmful to the cleansing process. Salt will calcify the mucoid plaque and the intestinal mucosa. It not only can ruin the Cleanse, but can cause permanent damage.

• If the stomach is sensitive to cayenne, just take one (1) capsule with every meal on Phase III and II, and don't take cayenne on Phase I. You can also eat a few bites of an apple to quench the flame of cayenne.

• We now recommend replacing chlorophyll and algae products with either Electro Life or Power-Up. These are incredibly effective products.

• Many people who have used cayenne with the herbs have actually doubled the amount of mucoid plaque removed, as compared to the other times they had done the Clean-Me-Out Program. Usually the dose was 3 high potency cayenne capsules each time the herbs were used. However, one should begin with a single capsule.

• **Throughout all phases of the Clean-Me-Out Program, we should always take Flora Grow.** Take 1 capsule at least 1 hour after the last set of herbs and at least 1/2 hour before bed. We have found that taking Flora Grow in this manner, prevents hunger and constipation after the Cleanse.

• When coming off the Cleanse, be sure you eat only organically grown produce. Not only is most of the commercially grown produce deficient in minerals and other nutrients, but it contains arsenic. Arsenic is used in herbicides and pesticides to kill bugs. Arsenic, like mercury and lead, is a deadly poison and is difficult to remove from the body. It has an accumulative effect. The older we become, the more prone we are to arsenic poisoning. I believe that over 30% of the American population is suffering to some degree from arsenic poisoning. From this day on, please eat only organically grown produce.

• **After any cleansing be sure to drink extra quantities of water.**

Before Starting the Clean-Me-Out Program

PLEASE DO THESE EASY pH [1] TESTS

Research confirms that the cause of most disease in America is always related to a deficiency of organic minerals. My own research has found that mucoid layers (plaque) are also caused by a lack of organic minerals. How do we lose our minerals? In order of most importance: 1. Eating too much acid-forming food. 2. Stressful emotions. 3. Overeating. 4. Infections from bacteria, parasites, yeast, fungus, and other microorganisms. 5. Metal toxicity such as mercury in teeth, arsenic in commercially grown food, etc. 6. Environmental pollution.

Quick summary of how most people drain their bodies of the alkaline minerals. Next to breathing and next to our heart beating, the next most important metabolic function our body performs is to maintain about 7.4 pH of the blood. If it cannot do this, then the body will become sick. Every metabolic function depends upon this delicate balance of pH.

The body has several ways it can rid itself of harmful acids. One of the most important ways, is through the bicarbonate buffer system. It is important to understand that this system cannot function without using organic minerals. The body takes these minerals and combines them with bicarbonate. Then it wraps this mixture around the acids and removes them out of the body. However, each time we eat acid-forming foods, we are ingesting potentially harmful acids and the body is then forced to lose valuable minerals. If our diet is too acid-forming or nutritionally deficient, then we cannot replenish these valuable elements. It is in this way that we gradually drain ourselves of minerals. When we lose our ready reserves of these alkaline minerals, then the body is forced to remove them from out of our own cells in order to maintain normal blood pH. This can cause radical metabolic imbalances known as disease.

---

1 pH: is a symbol used to measure acidity or alkalinity. Anything from 0 - 7, indicates acidity. The lower the number, the greater the acid level. Anything from 7 - 14, indicates alkalinity. The higher the number, the greater the alkaline level. It has to do with the potential hydrogen ion concentration.

If the blood pH begins to drop, and the alkaline mineral supply is low, then the body is forced to extract the needed minerals from anywhere it can get them. If the body removes sodium[2] from the stomach, then the stomach can no longer create hydrochloric acid. If it removes sodium from the bile, then the bile turns acid and not only will acid bile cause the formation of mucoid plaque, but every serious bowel disease (such as cancer, colitis, etc.) is based upon the bile being acid. If the body takes potassium from the heart, then heart disease can develop. If it removes minerals from the liver, then hundreds of problems can occur, including cancer. If it takes it from the bones, then osteoporosis and arthritis can occur, etc. This is the pattern that at least 96% of the American people have followed and are still following. It is primarily caused because of too much meat, dairy, junk food, pasta, pop, coffee, salt, alcohol, sugar, bread, and grains.

I have found that some people are too acid to do any kind of cleansing (except Phase III), fasting, or strenuous exercise without causing potential harm. The good news is that if we haven't drained ourselves too seriously, then it is easy to rebuild our supplies. Doing pH tests will indicate just how serious these depletions have become.

About 5% of vegetarians are too acid to do any rapid cleansing, fasting, or strenuous exercise. Up to 40% of meat-eaters are even more over-acid. Doing a simple pH test is very useful, for it will help us decide if we are healthy enough to safely do the Phase I of the Clean-Me-Out Program. (Even if we're over-acid, we can still cleanse slowly by using the Phase III.) The test will also help us to determine if we are in good health or just how fast we may be deteriorating and how we can improve our condition.

These tests are helpful in determining if we can do any deep cleansing, fasting, or strenuous exercising now, or if we must alkalize our bodies first.

How To Do the Three pH Tests
The following tests are not meant as instruction about pH.
They are only used to help determine if it is safe to cleanse.

The tools needed are pH papers, pencil, paper, and a lemon.

2 The body cannot use sodium chloride (table salt or sea salt). Sodium chloride is inorganic and is a poison to our bodies. It will help to drain organic sodium from our tissues.

119

I suggest pHydrion papers by Micro Lab - with 5.5 to 8.0 pH range. It is important to have pH paper that can be read in two-tenths increments. You may be able to get these pH papers at your local drug store or maybe at a health food store. (At the drug store you can expect to pay about $25.00. It should be less than half that amount at the health food stores that carry it (also available through Arise & Shine). When testing, it is important to get the paper very wet and read it between 10 and 30 seconds after first getting it wet. For the urine test, the paper can be placed in the stream of urine, or one can fill a container with urine and test it by dipping the paper into the fluid. Use just enough to get a reading. I know one person who uses about a quarter of an inch and his papers last a very long time. Some people use strips two inches long and that seems to be a waste. It's your choice.

Test One - The Saliva Test

Due to the unique characteristics of the mouth, such as its exposure to the air and bacteria, the mouth pH will not reach the normal levels of the blood. However, the saliva pH is a fairly accurate reflection of the pH in our cellular and extra cellular environment. The pH in the mouth should be about 6.4 to 7.

Directions: We do this test after we have had no food for at least two hours. Take a pH reading by wetting a strip of pH paper with saliva, and then holding it up to the color chart which is provided with the papers. Compare the wet paper to the nearest color and, presto! you have the pH reading. Now record it.

Note: People who are extremely sensitive to chemicals may wish to avoid putting the paper into the mouth. They can just spit into a cup and test it there.

Interpreting Test One - The Saliva Test:

6. or below = Possibly in a serious depleted condition and further testing is necessary. Indicates potential life-threatening danger when exercising or fasting.[3]

6.1 - 6.3 = Indicates depletion, but not dangerous. Further testing needed.

6.4 - 6.6 = Very good sign. Passed test one.

6.7 - 7.0 = Perfect for this part of the test.

7.1 or higher = Something may have interfered with the reading. It may be the thoughts about food, or it may indicate stress or excitement. Wait for about an hour and do the test again. If the reading remains the same, it indicates abnormal stress. It could be drugs, parasites, infections, emotions, etc. Stressful emotions are powerful enough to keep the body drained of minerals, no matter how good the diet is. Continue on with the other tests and keep a watchful eye for hints as to what is abnormal within.

Test Two - The Lemon Test

When we abruptly change the saliva pH with an acid lemon, the mouth should react quickly to this extremely acid condition by flushing alkalinity into the mouth. Within a few minutes after swallowing the lemon juice, we should have readings of 8 or above. If this does not occur it is another indication of a lack of alkaline minerals.

Directions: We do this test after we have had no food for at least two hours. (It can be done a few minutes after the Saliva Test, if you like.) Cut and squeeze the juice of ½ lemon into about 2 ounces of water, and drink. Swish in the mouth just a little bit as you drink it - no sweeteners. After swallowing lemon juice, wait for 60 seconds and then check saliva pH with the pH papers. Record reading on paper. Wait another 60 seconds and take another test and record. Do this every 60 seconds for a total of 6 times.

---

3 When we exercise we create lactic acid. Though the body can easily remove the lactic acid created by exercise through the lungs, its ability to do so can be inhibited when our bodies are already over-acid due to a lack of buffering minerals. In other words, when our bodies have lost the ability to maintain its normal alkaline pH, the body's metabolic function is decreased. It can't function as quickly nor as effectively as it should. Therefore, under already over-acid conditions, if the body is creating excess acids through exercise or stress, the body may not be capable of getting rid of the excess acids fast enough, and "boom" - the heart is flooded with excess acids and it stops. Many athletes and those who had a weak heart, have died for that reason. Saliva readings below 6.1 indicate this potential.

Interpreting Test Two - The Lemon Test:

Within six minutes, if the pH reading indicated an 8 or higher, then you passed the second test and most likely will pass the third, also. This would mean that we have ready alkaline reserves available, which is a very good indication that we are in good health.

If during the first test, the saliva reading was above 6.1, and we passed the second test (lemon), then it is safe to do Phase I (after completing Phase III). However, if the readings were on the low side, we should do all in our power to increase our alkaline reserve. By eating close to 100% alkaline-forming foods and using supplements which contain goat milk whey and beet crystals, we can usually rebuild our alkaline reserve quickly. By following these procedures during Phase III, a full alkaline reserve should be obtained by the time the Phase I begins. If this does not occur, it is because of one or more of the following reasons: 1. Alkaline minerals were drained to an extreme deficient state. 2. Emotional stress is high. 3. There is an acid-producing infection within the body. This could be parasites, bacteria, fungus, yeast, or viral. 4. There could be toxic metal poisoning within the body. This could be from mercury in teeth, arsenic from eating non-organic foods, lead and other metals from environment.

If readings of the lemon test were below 8 but above 7, we have also passed the second test, but the third test is necessary. This indicates that we have ready reserves of alkaline minerals, though not as much as we should. It says we'd better be careful and stay away from acid foods. It indicates that our body sometimes has to take minerals from our body organs, but not always. This means that we can do light cleanses, but we should not do Phase I or water fast yet, unless we pass the third test.

If readings are below 7, but higher than the reading taken in Test One - The Saliva Test, it would mean that there is some alkaline reserve left, but not much. It is necessary to take the third test and not likely that it will be passed. It is an indication that health may be in a serious condition. However, if stress is high, it could cause a misreading here; but even so, stress will weaken all bodily functions very quickly.

If the readings of the Lemon Test remain at or below the Test

One reading (before swallowing lemon), then this person is also in a seriously depleted condition. Fasting, cleansing (other than the Phase III), and strenuous exercise should not be done until the alkalinity is restored.

Test Three - The Urine Test

Urine pH changes quickly. It reveals how our bodies react to the food we ate the day before. When organic minerals are available in adequate amounts, urine pH will be acid after eating acid-forming foods. If we are deficient in organic minerals, then urine pH will be alkaline after eating acid-forming foods, because ammonia will be in the urine.

Directions: Choose a day when you can eat only acid-forming foods. (A list of acid and alkaline foods is available in the back of this book.) After eating only acid-forming foods for the entire day, the urine reading the following morning is very important. The very first voiding in the morning is the time to take this reading.

Interpreting Test Three - The Urine Test: (the next morning's urine test after eating acid-forming foods the day before):
6.8 or above = Body has no alkaline minerals to draw upon. The kidneys are forced to secrete ammonia directly into the urine. This occurs only after an extremely acid condition and when the body has no minerals to draw upon. The body uses ammonia to help compensate for the extreme acid accumulation. This is a state of alkalosis which is caused because of too much acid in the body.[4] This condition is serious and the odor of ammonia may be noticeable in the urine. This means that the body is unable to handle acids effectively and the liver and kidneys are operating in an emergency mode. Action should be taken immediately. No strenuous exercise and no cleansing (except Phase III) or fasting should be done. Diet needs to be changed quickly and emotional stress must be resolved. Gradually increase alkaline foods and decrease acid foods. Light exercise is beneficial, but do not run or exercise vigorously until saliva reading is above 6.1.

Note: How good a person feels is not an accurate indication of good health. If after eating acid-forming foods for one or more days and

4 Textbook of Medical Physiology, by Guyton, pg. 447.

the urine pH is above 6.8, then that person is physiologically sick - falling apart at the seams.

6.1 to 6.7 = Depletion is serious, but not dangerous. If the pH reading during Test One (The Saliva Test) was 6.1 or higher, and during Test Two (The Lemon Test), it was 7 or higher, it is OK to do all phases of the Clean-Me-Out Program; but it is necessary to drink mineral broths and/or carrot/celery juice and take organic electrolyte supplements while cleansing. Water fasting and strenuous exercise is not advised. If the lemon test reading was below 7, it is not advisable to do any cleansing except Phase III, until readings improve. This person should be on a crash program to bring the alkaline reserve back into balance. Read "How to replenish the alkaline minerals".

5.7 to 6.0 = Indication that alkaline minerals are available. The test has been passed, but it could be better.

5.6 or below = Good supply of minerals. Passed the test.

Note: These numbers are just a rough guideline, because each person will be choosing different acid foods and eating different amounts of them. It would be too difficult and complicated to measure just how acidic each person's intake was.

Summary of pH Tests

Indicators of serious mineral depletion and poor health regardless of how one feels:
>   1. Saliva pH between meals is below 6.1.
>   2. Lemon test does not reveal a pH above 7.
>   3. After eating acid-forming foods, the next morning's urine pH is above 6.1.
>   4. Smell of ammonia in urine.

Indicates good health - full reserve of alkaline minerals:
>   1. Saliva pH between meals is above 6.4.
>   2. Lemon test reveals 8 or above.
>   3. After eating acid-forming foods, the next morning's urine pH is 6 or below.

Explanation: Urine can only be acid if alkaline minerals are available to combine with the acids and remove the acids through the kidneys.

Saying this in another way may help: When we eat an acid meal for supper, the next morning our urine pH should be about 4.5 to 6, depending upon how acid the meal was and how much of it was eaten. If the body cannot obtain a low pH after acid meals the night before, it is because the body does not have any alkaline minerals to use. That means the body is stealing minerals from other parts of the body just to stay alive. People in this category often gain weight, because the body is diluting the acids with lymph and storing them, or they may lose weight and often suffer noticeable digestive disorders. This does not mean a healthy-looking person is free of these conditions. A person could be depleting their bones of calcium, their joints, stomach, liver, bile and muscles of sodium, etc. faster than the other two (obese & skinny) because they are unable to store acids in lymph or remove the acids out of the bowel.

If the morning urine pH readings after an acid meal are above a 6.8, then this is the worst situation of all. It means that this person has no alkaline reserve left. It indicates that the body is rapidly extracting minerals from organs and tissues, further depleting the system; and the kidneys are producing ammonia to alkalize the body just to keep it alive. People with these pH readings usually end up in the hospital and have serious chronic, and possibly degenerative, diseases.

These people can get sick when trying to alkalize their bodies. They must take it slowly and not try to alkalize too quickly. One exception: if they have AIDS, cancer, or some other degenerative disease, then they don't have time to alkalize gradually. They must act without delay, even though they will probably have a rough time of it. I recommend that these people find a doctor who understands the material in this book, and follow his or her advice. In any case, beginning Phase III immediately is recommended, for it will assist in removing acid-producing microorganisms from the bowel as well as removing metabolic stress. Drinking plenty of carrot/celery/apple juice and mineral broths is strongly recommended.

Those who did not pass the pH tests should stop eating acid foods, alkalize their bodies by eating mostly fruits, vegetables, mineral supplements (that are high in organic sodium, potassium, calcium, magnesium), and begin Phase III. After alkalizing and passing these tests, then it is safe to cleanse more deeply.

Note: After a healthy person eats alkaline-forming foods for a couple of days, the next morning's urine pH should be 7 or above. Everyone should strive for this.

Note: Whenever we are cleansing or fasting, our urine and saliva pH will drop, because the body is removing large amounts of acids.[5]

Miscellaneous Factors that can Influence pH

• Kidneys control pH. A problem concerning the kidneys can prevent a balanced pH.

• Breathing affects pH. Habitual shallow breathing can cause acidosis and may indicate a problem with the medulla.[6]

• High Altitude can cause a person to breathe at a faster rate, thereby increasing alkalinity.

• Lung damage or smoking can inhibit acids from being removed through the lungs.

• Stressful emotions create acids and cause increased acidity.[7]

• Parasite infections, fungal overgrowths, yeast infections, and bacterial overgrowths can create enough acidity to prevent a balanced pH.

HOW TO REPLENISH THE ALKALINE MINERALS

• Stop eating acid-forming foods.

• Eat only alkaline-forming foods such as fruits and vegetables.

• Drink carrot juice (organic).

• Take supplements that offer a quick supply of natural organic electrolyte minerals.

Note: For those who are extremely over-acid or over-alkaline, they could experience cleansing reactions if they attempt to replenish their alkaline minerals too fast. They should be doing Phase III as they go or eat a small amount of vegetarian acid-forming foods (like whole grains) to help keep them in balance.

---

5 For more good information about pH, read Your Health, Your Choice, and Correlative Urinalysis, by Ted M. Morter, Jr. B.S., M.A., D.C. B.E.S.T. Research, Inc. 1000 West Poplar, Rogers, Arkansas 72756,
1-800-874-1478.

6 Textbook of Medical Physiology, by Guyton, pg. 448.

7 Textbook of Medical Physiology, by Guyton, pg. 448.

HYPERSENSITIVE AND UNIVERSAL REACTORS

• Be sure to read the Check-off List and do the pH tests.

• For those who are extremely sensitive to foods, herbs, and practically everything else, who are "Universal Reactors", are very weak, very ill, very old, or are just plain nervous about cleansing or trying new herbs, it would be good to do a few tests before beginning Phase III. For example:

    1. Try only half (½) of a Chomper tablet alone. Wait a few hours and see how you feel. The next time try only one (1) and see. Do the same with Herbal Nutrition (or any herb unfamiliar to you, for that matter).

    2. When you make your first shake, try it with only half (½) teaspoon of psyllium and no bentonite (with the normal 4 oz. juice and 8 oz. water). The next one use both psyllium and bentonite, but both in tiny portions.

    3. Have only one or two (2)shakes per day, increasing portions until you're up to normal, or try a day with three (3) shakes (as per Phase III), but only half (½) portions.

• Following these gradual methods of taking herbs etc., will avoid any problems and help condition the body to handle larger doses. Slowly building up to larger doses makes it possible for people to get used to the herbs and then they can take the full-dose program.

• Increase at your own speed. All of the herbs are very natural, gentle, and safe, but you'll have more confidence if you increase slowly.

• After you've completed the normal Phase III (two meals per day) for a few weeks, then decide whether to do Phase II (one meal per day).

• You can alternate between Phase II and III, listening to your body's needs. Once comfortable with Phase II for a few days, you can then decide if you want to try Phase I (no meals).

• If you do Phase I, you may need to cut back a bit on the portions (psyllium, bentonite, herbs) for the first day, but still take five (5) shakes and five (5) sets of the herbs so you keep up your cleansing momentum.

Determining How Much Chomper
and Herbal Nutrition to Take

New Chomper: Now available in tablets (to eliminate the gelatin). These Chompers have less peristaltic action and no cayenne, and we can now take more. This will help eliminate a greater amount of the dreaded mucoid plaque more rapidly. Suggest starting with 5 tablets and watch the results. Check the section in the book about how to take Chomper.

New Herbal Nutrition: Has a special cellulase enzyme that increases the effectiveness of both Chomper and Herbal Nutrition when taken together. It is best to take the same amount of Herbal Nutrition as we do Chomper.

Important: Those who have used the original Chomper, but are now switching over to tablets, may find it is necessary to take 1 or 2 more tablets than the capsules. Since no two people are alike, each one must determine his own dosage of Chomper. Start with 3 capsules or 4 tablets, when taking the herbs. (With children and hypersensitive people, it is better to start out with small amounts, such as 1, and increase to 2 when they have been conditioned.) If stools seem too loose or runny, cut down the dosage by one. If the stools are hard or dry or if constipation has developed then increase the amounts until they are soft, yet formed. They should be soft enough to break apart when flushed. Sometimes, in serious cases of constipation, people have taken up to 30 or even 50 Chompers a day in order to break apart the constipated blockages. Remember, these herbs are food and can do no harm; however, we still need to proceed with caution because they are highly stimulatory. After the blockages are removed, we eliminate more easily and may need to cut back on the Chomper; but be alert, as you may need to increase them again at another time. It may also be necessary to decrease them again and later increase; however, this is usually not necessary.

How Much Herbal Nutrition to Take: As a general rule, those who are under 120 pounds should take 3 tablets or Herbal Nutrition, those who are between 120 and 170 pounds, should take 4; while those who are over 170 pounds should take 5.

Diarrhea? When using the original Chomper in gelatin capsules, about 5% of the people got diarrhea from taking only two. Cutting back to one, 5 times a day, would not make for an effective Cleanse, yet having diarrhea is not going to reveal that impressive mucoid material and is hard on the body. What do we do? First, try increasing the amount of bentonite and/or psyllium in the psyllium shake. Second, using the tablet form of Chomper (rather that the original capsules) should also help.

If you still have diarrhea, then try Chomper Enhancer, a formula I have designed just for situations like this. Everything remains the same except that we cut back on the Chomper to one or two, 5 times a day and take 1 or 2 teaspoons of Chomper Enhancer in a small glass of water at the same time we take the Chomper and Herbal Nutrition. It works very well. Chomper has a laxative effect and Chomper Enhancer has none. This condition is unlikely to occur with the new Chomper in tablets.

People Have the Greatest Results on Phase I: Many people feel better when on Phase I than they normally feel without cleansing. People who have fungus problems, such as yeast infections, or are extremely toxic, may not feel good while on Phase I. On this phase, these people can have such huge amounts of toxic matter trying to escape, that when it gets into the bloodstream, they feel terrible. I was one of these people and I certainly know what it is like. The first 10 cleanses I did, I had some rough times. (The first 9 were different cleanses, not the "Clean-Me-Out Program".) Alternating from one Phase to another will greatly help and can prevent this situation. However, the average person usually feels increased energy and alertness while on Phase I, or any of the other Phases. Often there will be ups and downs. I mean they may feel just fine for a while, then suddenly feel weak or tired for a few hours, and then feel good again. That is just the toxins being removed.

Example of the Pre-Cleanse *without* Liquid Minerals

6:30 AM Psyllium Shake	2:30 PM Herbs
8:00 AM Herbs	4:00 PM Psyllium Shake
9:30 AM Psyllium Shake	5:30 PM Herbs
11:00 AM Herbs	6:30 - 7:00 PM Dinner w/ Cayenne
12:00 - 12:30 Lunch w/ Cayenne	9:00 PM Herbs: Add a Chomper

When people get off schedule, it is OK to take the shake or eat one hour after the Herbs, but it is important to **wait at least one-and-a-half hours after the shake and two hours after eating to take the Herbs.** To make it easier, see the charts on page 136 and 137.

What to Eat While on the Pre-Cleanse (Phase III)

Absolutely No	Limited	OK
Bread	Beans	Fresh raw juice
Canned & frozen food	Cooked grains	Fruits
Chocolate	Honey	Millet
Cigarettes[1]	Popcorn	Potatoes
Coffee & Soft Drinks	Maple Syrup	Raw vegetables
Dairy & Eggs		Salads
Distilled vinegar		Sprouts
Foods cooked with oil		Steamed vegetables
Fried foods, margerine		Supplements[2]
Meat, fish, birds		Vegetable soup
Nuts & Seeds		
Salt, sugar		
Store-bought cereals		
Tofu and Soy products		
Wheat products		

NOTE: "YEAST END" If we suspect Candidiasis, E-Coli, salmonella, other harmful bacteria or fungus have gained control in the bowel, we should take Yeast End; however, it must be used with caution as its effect is to eliminate unwanted organisms, and a toxic reaction can occur. It is important to build up the intestinal flora using Flora Grow for 1 to 2 weeks prior to the use of Yeast End. Then take Yeast End

---

[1] If an addiction (like cigarettes or coffee) is so ingrained that you feel too discouraged to cleanse, at least decrease your intake of these toxins on the Pre-Cleanse. Then try to quit entirely while on Phase I. This would be better than not cleansing at all. After cleansing, we find we can change our habits much more easily. Herbal Nutrition has helped many people overcome the addiction to smoking.

[2] Nutritional supplements are OK, as long as they are natural and not synthetic, such as found in drug stores. However, we should not take things such as Homozon, Duetrosulfazyme, or anything that affects peristalsis.

once a day as indicated above for the first 2 weeks to help control yeast found in the throat and/or stomach. Then increase to 1 in the morning and evening for 2 more weeks. Yeast End may also be dissolved in the mouth to help eliminate yeast there. More extreme candida infestations may require up to 3 bottles. Children's dosage is half the potency of the adult. If severe diarrhea occurs for more than 2 days, discontinue.

TESTIMONIALS

The following are true reports from people who used the Clean-Me-Out Program.

I'm Pregnant !!!!!

My health has generally been good, however 2 years ago I was diagnosed with endometriosis and told I would not conceive. Doctors began with a 9 month course of birth control to be followed by Danocryn, which I refused. Symptoms worsened so I turned to wholistic treatments with herbs and magnets. Shortly after that I was introduced to the "Clean-Me-Out" Program by Charles B. I completed it last March with great success. My whole life changed for the better. Since then I have continued to cleanse and eat raw foods. The great news is that yesterday I found out I'm pregnant! I have had no morning sickness. I truly believe I got pregnant because I cleaned out a lot of old toxins that were preventing me from carrying a baby in a safe environment. I feel so blessed to have done the cleanse. I feel it's the greatest gift I have ever given myself. I have a health and beauty aids business (for 7 years now) with approximately 600 "regular" female clients. I want to promote the cleanse to all of them. My closest friends are already convinced of the benefits and 6 of them are ready to begin the program...

As far as benefits of the cleanse, to name a few...I have more energy than I know what to do with. I wake up clear headed, don't need coffee, I do skin brushing instead. I'm not sleepy after meals. I feel light and energized. I watch very little T.V. because I can't sit still that long. Our grocery bill is less than half of what it was before. I'm making everything fresh so I don't concern myself about preservatives. I feel satisfied at each meal because I'm a conscious eater now. I don't snack because I don't have cravings. I feel healthier because my food is moving through me at a faster pace. And I feel younger, which is terrific! Christine D., Spring Valley, California.

Immune System Restored

I am now 23 years old and for the past eight years I have suffered from a total immune system breakdown, beginning with ulcerate colitis, and heightening to relapsing poly-choncritis, which is the immune system attacking and eating away cartilage in the body. Other symptomatic problems I experienced; severe body itching, terrible facial acne, liver and digestion dysfunction, hair loss, low energy level... All "western" medical philosophies dictated I would have to endure this my entire life. I refused to accept that.

The past eight years of mental battles, vegetarianism, acupuncture, and soul searching have resulted in about 80% recovery. Recently, Marie M., an Arise & Shine Distributor, gave me a copy of Cleanse And Purify Thyself. After reading it, I realized why all of my health problems occurred in the first place. Years of McDonald's, Jack in the Box, and other poisonous foods of that sort, along with continual year round doses of antibiotics had devitalized my digestion, assimilation and evacuation; thus decimating my body.

I immediately started on a cleanse; a two week pre-cleanse followed by a one week fast. During the pre-cleanse, all my colitis symptoms (constant bloody diarrhea evacuation) which had been gone for so long, returned: Healing crisis. During the first three days of the fast, I felt very sluggish and nauseated. On the fourth day my energy level shot up to the level it was as a child; my nose started growing back where the cartilage had been lost; and my itching stopped. Performing two colemas a day during the fast, I evacuated at least 15 feet of black ropy impacted fecal matter, shaped like the colon and intestines.

For the past three years, I have itched myself, especially my legs, bloody almost every single night! Since my cleanse, I have not itched one single time! My energy is increasing every day and I love it... I now see that no matter how much you take care of yourself, you cannot achieve total health unless your body is clean and pure. Sincerely, Chad M., Santa Monica, California.

Recovered From The Deadly Affects of Medical Radiation

One health practitioner said that one of her clients, "...who had bladder cancer three or so years ago and they over radiated her and she had no control over her bowels. They said it'd be that way for the rest of her life. After one week on the Cleanse her bowels are moving on their own in the morning and no uncontrollable diarrhea." Catherine, Tucson.

Bone Cancer Pain Reduced

A man in terrible pain from bone cancer came to me. After his first Cleanse he reported, "Rich, at least 75% of the pain just disappeared."

Critically High Blood Pressure Back To Normal

One lady in California told me after she did the Cleanse, " I had very dangerous high blood pressure for over a year. Nothing the doctors did ever helped my condition, but on the sixth day of the "Clean-Me-Out Program, I went back to the doctor for a check up. He was shocked to discover my blood pressure was normal." L.J.

What Goes In Doesn't Always Come Out

A lady in Idaho reported that ever since she could remember she had a hard lump in her abdomen. About half way through the Cleanse she had a very strange sensation just below her stomach. She drove home as fast as she could and soon passed a hard piece of material about 6 or 7 inches long and about two inches thick. She cleaned it off and when her husband looked at it, he hit it on the toilet and it sounded almost like metal. Then he hit it hard and broke it. Inside were multi-colors. When she saw that she instantly knew that it was from all the color crayons that she had eaten when she was about five years old. From then on the hard lump was gone. She was so impressed with the Cleanse that she had perhaps 50 or more people that she knew take the Cleanse.

Cancer Pain Gone - Plus Happy Side Benefits

T. Miles from San Francisco had Lymphoma cancer under his right arm. Talk of pain! After the Clean-Me-Out Program, the pain was completely gone.

And a Cripple Lady Walks Normally Again

"For the last seven years, I have been dealing with a steadily increasing amount of pain in my right hip. For the last six months, the pain had become so great that I was using a cane regularly outside of the house. X-Rays showed that the cartilage had worn off the head of the femur. An infection had also developed. The nerves at the head of the femur were telling my brain to immobilize the right leg. In spite of many different types of therapy to reverse the steady downward spiral, nothing seemed to turn the gradual decline around. The different therapies I tried included...chiropractic treatments, therapeutic massage, nutrition, exercise... homeopathy, yoga, as well as colon cleansing using Dr. Jensen's program... Approximately ten weeks ago, I started using the herbal products from Arise & Shine in preparation for a one week colon Cleanse. I took Herbal Nutrition and Chomper six weeks before beginning the Cleanse. For the colon Cleanse, I did everything suggested in the book, "Cleanse & Purify Thyself," On the second day of the Cleanse, approximately 50% of the pain left my body and I stopped using the cane at that time. On the third day of the Cleanse, I did a little yoga with my yoga students for the first time in over a year. They were watching me with their mouths open because their most recent experience of me was seeing a person move with great agony and pain. Marie M.

Children Benefit Too

A mother wrote, "My six year old, after weeks of the old Pre-Cleanse and mostly raw foods, passed a six inch chunk of old, blackish-brown, dried mucoid matter with striations... on the very first day of the new Pre-Cleanse. Proof that, 'Yup! he did need it too.' We're both more excited now that we're seeing results. We'll be back in touch post-cleanse... Glad you're there. Thanks. Pamela"

A Lady From Canada Wrote

"I tried it. On the second day I could not believe how good I felt and the stuff that came out of me looked like the gunk when an alien starts disintegrating." Mrs. D. Urgwhart,"

Serious Headaches Vanish

"I have had the most excruciating headaches anyone would ever have for many years now. Do you think that you can help me?" I could see that her elimination systems were far from normal and her body was accumulating toxic debris. Soon she was on the Pre-Cleanse and after 10 days went on the full Cleanse. She began to lose some unnecessary weight and before the Cleanse was over she told me the headaches were, for the first time in years, completely gone. She became vibrant and outgoing and started to enjoy life in a way that had been impossible up to that time.

The Average Testimony

People report more energy (the most common), feel better, feel closer to God, pain is gone, skin looks better, lumps disappeared, have better control over the emotions and feel happier.

ALKALINE-ASH FOODS

Alfalfa Sprouts	Cherries
Beets & Greens	Figs, Fresh
Broccoli	Grapefruit
Brussel Sprouts	Grapes
Cabbage	Lemons
Carrots	Leeche Nuts
Cauliflower	Limes
Celery	Mangoes
Collard Greens	Oranges
Cucumbers	Pineapple
Dulse	Apples
Green Beans	Apricots
Green Limas	Blackberries
Green Peas	Blueberries
Green Soy Beans	Nectarines
Kale	Peaches
Kelp	Pears
Leaf lettuce	Raspberries
Mushrooms	
Mustard Greens	Apricots, Dried
Okra	Avocado
Onions	Bananas
Parsley	Dates
Peppers	Figs, Dried
Potatoes	Raisins
Parsnips	
Radishes	Cantaloupe
Rhubarb	Honeydew
Rutabagas	Watermelon
Sauerkraut	
Spinach	Misc.
Sprouts	Vinegar,
Squash	Cider
Turnip Greens	Lima Beans
Tomatoes	Maple Syrup
Water Cress	Molasses
Yams	Fresh Corn

Exceptions: Spinach, citrus & pineapple. Eat small amounts & only if citrus & pineapple are fully ripe. Note: All foods become acid when sugar is added.

ACID-ASH FOODS

Alcohol
Aspirin
Barley, Pearled
Bread, Wheat
Cake
Cereals, All
Chickpeas
Chocolate
Coffee
Corn
Corn starch
Cranberries
Eggs & All Dairy Products
Grains except millet
Honey
Legumes
Lentils
Niacin
Mustard
Nuts
Oatmeal
Pasta
Plums & Prunes
Pepper, Black
Rice
Seeds
Soda Crackers
Soft Drinks
Sugar
Tea, Black
Vinegar, Distilled
Vitamin C
Wheat Bran
Wheat Germ
Wheat Products
Fruits - canned, glazed or sulfured

All Animal Products-includes Birds, Fish and Sea Foods. On Acid days, limit coffee, pop, cola or black tea to 2 cups.

Long pH Test: Contact Arise & Shine for instructions.

135

PHASE II OR III CLEANSE RECORD

Using Liquid Minerals

Day of the Week							
Record your own times.	Day 1	Day 2	Day 3	Day 4	Day 5	Day 6	Day 7
6:30 Shake[1]							
7:45 Minerals[2]							
8:00 Herbs[3]							
9:30 Shake							
10:45 Minerals							
11:00 Herbs							
12:30 Shake or Lunch[4]							
2:15 Minerals							
2:30 Herbs							
4:00 Shake							
5:15 Minerals							
5:30 Herbs							
6:30 Supper[4]							
8:45 Minerals							
9:00 Herbs with Extra Chomper							
10:00 Flora Grow							

1 Shake = 1 or 2 Tablespoons Bentonite, 2 - 4 oz. juice, 8 oz. water. Add 2 teaspoons of Psyllium, shake and drink, then drink *another* 8 oz. of water. Be sure to wait at least 1-1/2 hours after Shake before taking herbs!

2 Liquid Minerals = About 1-2 Tablespoons per dose (depending on body weight), with 1 or 2 oz. juice

3 Herbs = 3 or more Chomper & 3 or more Herbal Nutrition. Optional: 1 Cayenne and/or 2-4 Blue Green Algae or Chlorophyll

4 Meals = Alkaline Diet, preferably raw fruit or raw vegetables. One meal per day on Phase II. Two meals per day on Phase III. Choose which shake to replace with a meal. Optional: With vegetable meals, One Cayenne and 2-4 Blue Green Algae or Chlorophyll

NOTE: Feel free to adjust the times to suit *your* schedule.

PHASE I CLEANSE RECORD
Using Liquid Minerals

Day of the Week							
Record your own times.	Day 1	Day 2	Day 3	Day 4	Day 5	Day 6	Day 7
6:30 Shake[1]							
7:45 Minerals[2]							
8:00 Herbs[3]							
9:30 Shake							
10:45 Minerals							
11:00 Herbs							
12:30 Shake							
1:45 Minerals							
2:00 Herbs							
3:30 Shake							
4:45 Minerals							
5:00 Herbs							
6:30 Shake							
7:45 Minerals							
8:00 Herbs with Extra Chomper							
9:00 Flora Grow							

1 Shake = 1 or 2 Tablespoons Bentonite, 2 - 4 oz. juice, 8 oz. water. Add 2 teaspoons of Psyllium. Shake and drink quickly then follow with *another* 6-8 oz. of water! Be sure to wait at least 1-1/2 hours after Shake before taking herbs and *drink plenty of water!*

2 Liquid Minerals = About 1-2 Tablespoons per dose (depending on body weight), with 1 or 2 oz. juice

3 Herbs = 3 or more Chomper & 3 or more Herbal Nutrition. Optional: One Cayenne and/or 2-4 Blue Green Algae or Chlorophyll
    NOTE: Feel free to adjust the times to suit *your* schedule.

Index

Headaches
    during Cleanse, 67
    vanish after Cleanse, 125
Health
    of American People, 6-7
    professionals, 4, 104
Health Freedom, perserving, 108-109
Heart
    attack, 98
    cayenne for, 98-99
    pounding of, 98
Herbal Nutrition
    herbs in, 42-44
    history and development, 25-26
    taking on Cleanse, 52, 128-129
    vitamins and minerals in, 26
Herbs
    directions for taking, 52, 128-129
    for enemas, 63-64
    for immune system, 104
    in Chomper, 22, 40-41
    in Herbal Nutrition, 25, 42-44
    taken separately from Shake, 101
    versus drugs, 102
High Blood Pressure
    normal after Cleanse, 133
Hunger, while on the Cleanse, 26, 99
Hydrochloric Acid, 69

Immune System
    cleansing and herbs for, 104
    breakdown of, 10-11
    effect of radiation therapy on, 13
    restored, 132
Implantation of Flora Grow
    directions for, 58
    success of, 87
Intestines
    cleansing of, 10-11, 28
    drawings of, 29-30
    harmfulness of, 105-106
    length of, 11
    nourishment assimilated in, 31
    peristaltic action of, 32
    irradiated foods, 105
    harmfulness of, 105-106

Jensen, Dr. Bernard, 10
    Iridology Chart, 34-36

Jesus, Master
    Gospel of Peace, 14-16, 70-71, 83-85,
        112
Junk food, effects of, 73-76, 86
Just, Adolf, *Return to Nature*, 106-107

Life Force
    and dead foods, 81
    for health, 80
Liquid Minerals
    directions for taking, 48
    for better results on Cleanse, 50
    source of, 110-111
    use in cleansing, caution, 48
    value of, 47
Lymph, 11-12

Malnutrition, 10, 12
Meat/Meat Eaters
    cancer and, 31
    eating after Cleanse, 102-103
    effects of, 9, 68-69, 71-72, 119
    negative feelings and, 17
    preparation for Cleanse, 102
    reactions during Cleanse, 55
Menstrual periods
    changes during Cleanse, 100-101
Milk
    effect of cow's, 68-69
    raw goat's milk, 69
Mucoid Layers/Substance
    and parasites/worms, 17
    creation of, 9
    effect on body, 10
    effect on emotions, 16, 17
    effect on nerves, 33
    examination and length of, 11, 24
    in intestinal tract, 11-12, 27
    peristalsis affected by, 9

Natural Healing, 4, 7,
    of pneumonia, 10
Negative Energy,
    thoughts & feelings, 13, 17
Nerves, improvement of nerve flow, 33
Nutrients, absorption of, 32, 80

Obesity
    after Cleanse, 92
    effect on lymphatic system, 33-34